Funny Farm

Dr. Eileen A. Schweickert

BMS
Book Marketing Solutions
Traverse City, Michigan

Funny Farm
by Dr. Eileen A. Schweickert

Copyright © 2007 by Dr. Eileen Schweickert

Cover art by Bud Schweickert
Page and cover design by BMS

All rights reserved. No part of this book may be reproduced or transmitted in any form or by any means, electronic or mechanical, including photocopying, recording, or by any information storage retrieval system without written permission from the publisher.

Published by BMS
An imprint of Book Marketing Solutions
10300 E. Leelanau Court
Traverse City, MI 49684

sales@BookMarketingSolutions.com
www.BookMarketingSolutions.com

Printed in the United States of America

Schweickert, Eileen A.
   Funny farm / Eileen A. Schweickert. -- Traverse City, Mich. : Book Marketing Solutions, c2007.
     p. ; cm.
     ISBN: 978-1-934792-01-8
     1. Multiple sclerosis--Patients--Biography. 2. Laughter--Therapeutic use. 3. Wit and humor--Psychological aspects. 4. Adjustment (Psychology) 5. Schweickert, Eileen A.--Health. I. Title.

RC377 .S38 2007
362.1/96834/0092--dc22   0710

This book is available at
www.ReadingUp.com

Dedication

This book is dedicated to my Father, George Henry Schweickert, Jr., who died on January 3, 2007. My Dad was the personification of the word "gentleman." He was a peace loving man who dedicated his life to his family and his country. He taught me that you can make a lot happen if you polish a dream with plenty of elbow grease.

Acknowledgements

Since this is my first book, I needed a lot of help pulling this project off. My mother, Ruth Schweickert, was kind enough to provide a first edit of the book and cleaned it up pretty well.

The folks at Book Marketing Solutions have been wonderful teachers. I especially appreciate all the time Denise Glesser has devoted to this endeavor. My formal editor, Ilene Stankiewicz, did a smooth job of polishing up my work without detracting any of its essence. She was painless to work with.

The cover art is my brother Bud Schweickert's creation. I had a blast working on the project with him.

My brother, Chuck, and all the rest of my extended family members and friends, have been rooting support people during my illness, as well as during the writing of this book. Thank you for not writing me off when I got withdrawn and surly. I especially thank Cowboy Bob Brown for taking on my chores when I am unable to do them. And blessings for my darling Flora, my former practice partner, for having the strength and dedication to continue with the dream when she had to go on alone. This book is for you!

My husband, Dan, was gracious about all the meals missed because I was writing, and never tired of hearing me read parts of the book aloud to him. His support during this most difficult period literally saved my life. I love you!

Contents

Introduction	11
Chapter 1 Why Bucking Bulls?	19
Chapter 2 Myths about Bull Riding and Bull Riders	33
Chapter 3 Heifers on Board	43
Chapter 4 Baffler's Syndrome	51
Chapter 5 Picasso and Dali	59
Chapter 6 Waiting for Bonnie Blue	67
Chapter 7 Chicken Rancher Maile	75
Chapter 8 Laying an Egg	83

Chapter 9 Breakfast in Bed	89
Chapter 10 The Grand Procession	95
Chapter 11 Cali Rae	101
Chapter 12 Bloody Rooster	111
Chapter 13 The Day the Poop Wagon Attacked	123
Chapter 14 Cowgirls Love Trucks	133
Chapter 15 Black Gold	139
Chapter 16 Stomping Chickens	147
Chapter 17 Newcomers	157

Chapter 18 Mornings with Martha	163
Chapter 19 Turtling	169
Conclusion	175
Mahalo	179
About the Author	181

Introduction

I suspect you'd like to know a little about me in order to have a frame of reference for this collection of stories. Then you can decide whether to ante up the purchase price for this book. If you want a hint about this book's flavor, picture something written by Erma Bombeck if she had decided to become a cattle rancher. I am a stock contractor and I raise bucking bulls.

I was formerly an overworked, underpaid, small

Dr. Eileen A. Schweickert

town family doctor but had to give up that line of work due to a nasty disease called multiple sclerosis. This is a collection of tales about my experiences along the journey between these two careers. It is also about not giving up, no matter what bad things happen to you. I've learned that you have to remember you are still living till you're not. Because, then you're really dead. Until the big "The End," there is still life to be enjoyed.

A bit about my history. Growing up, I was a military brat, traipsing around the world with my bomb expert dad who was in the Air Force, my stay-at-home mom, and my two younger brothers. We ended up in Hawaii on the north shore of Oahu, and I attended a rural high school there in the tiny, sugar plantation town of Waialua. I was one of about eight white or "haole" kids in my graduating class.

In my 20s, I was blessed to be able to spend my hours in study at the Manoa campus of the University of Hawaii. My 30s led me through medical school in California and into a re-

Introduction

warding career in family medicine in northern Michigan. Along the way I married, divorced, and ever the optimist, remarried. My 40s were spent teaching medicine and climbing the ladder of academia. As my 50s rolled around, I settled on being that small town doctor I'd always wanted to be. I left teaching and joined my career partner, and moved into private medical practice. And life was good. I loved my work. I expected to slog on till I was about 70. My home life was happy. I told people I never imagined that life could be so fulfilling. And then things started to fall apart.

A year into my new practice endeavor, I began having a wide range of neurological problems. As the severity of the symptoms increased, I struggled to make adaptations in my work schedule to accommodate my shadowy disabilities. My problems waxed and waned. I thought I was working too hard and sleeping too little. I thought most of what was going on was probably in my head. I tried to ignore what was happening, and I worked more. Finally, after a frightening crescendo of symptoms, my hus-

Dr. Eileen A. Schweickert

band and I sought professional medical help. I was told that my diagnosis most likely was *relapsing remitting multiple sclerosis*. As the words "multiple sclerosis" came from the neurologist's mouth, I felt my world start to implode.

For the next six months, I attempted all kinds of schedule and responsibility alterations, grasping at the hope that I could continue my practice. My work was my heart and soul. But limiting my practice proved almost more stressful than working 60-70 hour weeks. Finally, in February 2004, after a particularly terrible fall, I went on a medical leave of absence. It was the first time in my adult life that I was not working. The impact was psychologically devastating.

My purpose in life was gone. I sat home and mourned. I seriously contemplated suicide. My husband, Dan, who had been semiretired, went back to work. We decided to move to lessen his commute to his new job. We had been planning to move out of our small town and into the

Introduction

countryside for retirement, and now I needed a house that did not have a second floor so I could get around more easily. We searched and found a property that met all our new requirements.

Prior to the onset of my illness, we had been dreaming of starting a hobby farm ranching bucking bulls. Yes, bulls, as in bull riding, like in rodeo. My husband somehow realized that I needed a project to tie myself to in order to have a reason to go on. So he decided that we'd activate our retirement plan and I would be chief rancher. Although everyone we knew thought we were nuts, we bought a parcel of land off an unpaved country road, with a house that met my needs, and started a whole new life. We downshifted big time.

I was accustomed to working long days. My practice had been large and my patients' needs diverse. I had also been teaching medical students and residents, participating in community service endeavors, and doing lots of work related travel. I sat on the National Board of

Dr. Eileen A. Schweickert

Directors of the American Medical Women's Association, the organization that was established by female physicians when the American Medical Association did not allow women doctors membership. I had been one busy gal. Now I sat looking out on my acreage with nothing to do. I felt like my life was over.

I could not walk independently. My vision problems made reading impossible. I slept 12 to 18 hours out of 24. When awake, about all I could do was watch television. Luckily, I am easily bored and there is nothing more boring than daytime television. Oprah has some interesting stuff on, but she and Dr. Phil can't compete with what I'd been up to myself before I became disabled. While I still had a desperate need to be emotionally and mentally active, my physical limitations seemed an overwhelming barrier.

But my husband, who kept me plugged into our dream and the beauty of the land around me, contributed to my healing by not letting me give up. Slowly, my body stabilized. With the

Introduction

help of friends and loved ones, and support of organizations like the MS Society, I found treatments for my illness and solace for my broken spirit. As we learned about ranching, we found our sanity and I began to heal. First I got better mentally. Then my physical body started to get stronger. I believe the land and our animals have literally have saved my life. And we have had some great and crazy adventures along the way. This is the story of how two city slickers started a bucking bull breeding program and how our animals saved my butt.

Humor has been one of the constant elements in our daily adventures. And though disability and illness are not usually funny topics, for me, when I started to laugh again, I started to live. My husband, bless his heart, never stopped laughing even when things looked pretty bleak. In the hope that there might be others who can benefit from our crazy experiences, or at least use a good laugh, I share our story with you. My animals have given full permission to freely discuss our adventures in hopes that

Dr. Eileen A. Schweickert

maybe other critters will have an easier time breaking in their humans. I have tried to format these tales so that they would be suitable for readers of all ages, and can be shared by being read aloud.

Chapter 1

Why Bucking Bulls?

A question people are always asking me is why, of all things, are you raising bucking bulls? I guess the best short answer is that I have a genetic inclination towards extreme sports, but my age and Pennsylvania Dutch heritage have yielded a body fit for just one thing, being a stock contractor. So here I am. Keep reading for the long answer.

My father was a career military man. He enlisted in the service at age 17. He was an explosives technician and spent a good part of his life mucking about in Southeast Asia, taking bombs apart in the Agent Orange dripping jungle. My youngest brother lives on a sailboat in the Virgin Islands and is a kiteboarder. His idea of a high time is weathering hurricanes while moored in a mangrove swamp. My middle brother lives amidst a pack of six pit bulls and he is not Cesar Milan. His dogs regularly escape, fight, or just cause injury and mayhem by virtue of their number and size. My mom can't visit him without wearing hockey pads; she gets knocked down at least once every time we're on the phone when she calls from his house.

I have always been an animal lover, but we never had big animals while I was growing up due to our frequent moves, the result of Dad's military service. Dan and I began our married life with three cats, then added a potbellied pig and a dog before I became ill. We began to follow professional bull riding around the time it became a standalone sport and the Professional Bull Riders (PBR) Tour was formed. We

Why Bucking Bulls?

noticed some of the same indications of intelligence in these specially bred bovines, pitted against the top cowboy riders, that we'd noted in our pot bellied pig. We became fascinated by these special cattle.

Since my childhood days visiting my grandfather's family's dairy farm in New York state, I'd longed to settle in the country and have a bit of land. Dan and I thought that when I retired from my practice and could move "off call" and out of town, we'd try raising some bucking stock ourselves. But I became ill and Dan went back to full-time employment at a job located 50 miles south of where we had been living. So we decided to buy a place that met my mobility needs, moved us closer to his job, and provided the setting we needed to start our ranch. Originally, the ranch part was still a "down the road" dream.

When I first stopped working, I was a trashed. I could not walk without a walker or cane, and my vision problems prevented me from reading. I was angry and depressed to the point of thinking about ways to kill myself. But I get bored easily, and very soon was I was bored with being self-absorbed. Dan used every opening he could to try to occupy me with our new life and keep me moving forward. First I read farming magazines and cruised Web sites about ranching. Then I started walking about our acreage. Next thing I knew, we bought some miniature guard donkeys.

My next step was talking an established stock contractor into selling us two prime heifers with incredible pedigrees. I think the stock contractor felt sorry for me, and I probably should feel guilty because he just about gave me those girls, but what the heck! Someday I'll do something equally nice for someone else. Now we actually had cattle! And it was my job to tend them.

I do my chores spread out over as much time as my body requires, taking breaks when I need them. These two heifers have been great companions in my recovery. They are fine, high-spirited, gorgeous creatures. They're intelli-

Why Bucking Bulls?

gent, and when you watch them run and turn and buck, you take in a sight that makes you glad to be a fellow living critter.

The environment I spend my days in isn't too shabby, either. I'm outside in the fresh air. Most of the country lanes in the counties surrounding my ranch are lined with huge, old maple trees. In the winter they look like a talented artist's charcoal drawings against the stark, white snow. In summer, these giants leaf out in multiple shades of green, forming an umbrella across the roads to shade the lanes from the heat. They provide a welcome vertical counterpoint to the horizontal lines of fields filled with corn and soybeans.

Much of my healing has come from slowing down the pace of my life. As I work, I watch the small birds sunning themselves in the trees, enjoying a break from the icy cold. I too feel the sun warm the backs of my black tights just like it does their dark wings. It feels good. In the early 1900s, there was a movement in psychiatry to incorporate beauty and work in

Dr. Eileen A. Schweickert

treatment for mental ills. Dr. James D. Munson, superintendent of the Regional State Psychiatric Hospital here in Traverse City during that era, was one of this theory's proponents. Patients were encouraged to work on a farm that was a part of the institution and provided for much of its needs. Physical activity in a pleasant setting was believed to be soothing and have healing properties. I believe Dr. Munson was right.

People frequently ask me about the improvement in my health over the last several years. I have to attribute a good bit of the improvement in my well-being to the therapeutic effect of my beautiful surroundings. Our land is gorgeous. There are open expanses of pasture and forested areas, each with its own natural population of animal life. We're trying to share the land with these indigenous creatures. We have encountered a wide array of bird life, rabbits, raccoons, toads, coyotes, and this summer we even saw some bear tracks in the back pasture. At my current pace, I have time to notice all these things.

Why Bucking Bulls?

There is not much that can match the sight of a male cardinal feasting on dried berries on a bush against the fresh, pure white of new snow. When you can stand and look down your road into the dusky twilight and not be disturbed by another human soul for half an hour to an hour at a time, you have time to breathe deeply. And then, when you do, you smell fresh cut hay, not car exhaust. The beauty comes flooding into you with multisensory lushness. Some times I feel drunk on it.

I think this slower pace has had the biggest effect on quieting my discombobulated immune system. Additionally, I have tried to feed my body the healthiest, locally grown food I can find. The less it has traveled before it reaches my mouth, the higher I believe its nutrient value. I try to eat whole foods, avoiding processed, fake food and things like genetically modified organisms (GMOs) and trans fats. I eat little meat. I don't drink pop and I do drink a lot of fresh water. I sleep more than I did before.

Dr. Eileen A. Schweickert

I listen to music much of the time but I don't read the newspaper regularly or watch the news every night. I read books and magazines voraciously, as my vision allows. Luckily, my local library has a great collection of large print books. My library card is one of my most prized possessions. When I can't read, I listen to books on tape.

I've also learned some tai chi from my mother and have added this to some yoga based stretching that I do every day. The tai chi especially seems to have helped me regain control of my balance and relearn to walk with a more normal gait. When the weather allows, I do my morning tai chi routine outside so I can feel the wind and sun, hear the birds, and smell the earth as I do it. I spend as much of each day outside as I can.

Even when a day is starting out poorly, with a lot of pain or other difficulty, I've learned that if I can just get outside, things immediately start to improve. So, on a really crummy day, I don't worry about dishes or laundry or

Why Bucking Bulls?

making the bed. I just think about getting outside, even if it's just to sit. What will usually happen after I sit for awhile, is that I slowly begin to feel better and have the inclination to move some, perhaps only to bend over and to pull a few weeds. Once I do this, however, I may be up to feeding the chickens, and then I'm on my way. I am certainly not advocating that everyone with MS start a farm, or even that anyone will find this same recipe works for them. But finding ways to increase the variety and quality of pleasurable sensory experiences that flow across one's senses surely will help healing.

My fiercest battle is with pain. I have pain all the time. It never abates. Sometimes it is better, sometimes it is worse. For the first year or so, I thought there would be some drug out there that would take it away. At least for periods of time. This never happened. And I was lucky in that my physicians were willing to use all types of medication in treating me. I was not perceived as a "drug seeker" like some chronic pain patients are. I was resistant initially to using narcotic medications. But I finally decided that they were a better choice than suicide and I never took them during the time I was seeing patients. I was concerned about the appearance of any impairment in the event of a mistake or bad outcome.

Yet even narcotic pain medications have not been able to relieve all my pain. For a couple of years, pain ruled my life. Gradually I learned to use other methods to make life bearable. One of the keys to pain control in chronic pain syndromes involves using external distraction to shift a person's focus from pain to something more pleasant. I've found both physical activity and pleasant surroundings to be useful in this way. What I've discovered is that the endorphins released during movement are a powerful ally. When I do tai chi, I get an immediate reduction in pain. When I get busy mucking out sheds, I forget to focus on what my legs feel like and my pain is better. Or at least I tolerate it better.

This may be a convoluted answer, but as best as

Why Bucking Bulls?

I can relate, this is why I breed bucking bulls. And we certainly have quite a list of characters here on the 4B Ranch. I'll introduce you to them, so you will know who I'm referring to as I tell you about my experiences. By the way, the 4B is short for Bluewater Bay Bucking Bulls, and this is the name of our endeavor. The name pays tribute to all the gorgeous waterways we have in northern Michigan. Dan is an Acadian waterman by birth, and I have the water as my "amakua," or thing that speaks for my soul. The only water we actually have on the ranch is found in mud puddles when we get a hard rain, though, so our name is also a bit of a take-off on some of the high-sounding titles frequently bestowed upon developments, cottages, and resorts in this neck of the woods.

First on my list is my husband, Dan, who is also quite a character. He must be, if he agreed to this ranching idea! Dan was born in Detroit. He's half French Acadian and half Czechoslovakian. His father worked in the auto plants during Detroit's boom years. Dan is trained as

Dr. Eileen A. Schweickert

an old school mechanic and knows car, snowmobile, and marine guts.

When we moved to the 4B, our zoo already included several pets. There was Maile Jane, a young beagle, and two rescue cats—an orange tom, named Tiki the Toilet Weasel, and Pintail O'Reilly. Tiki was head of rodent control and Pintail is retired (she is somewhere between 13 and 30 years old). Our indoor brood has been anchored by the critter that runs our lives, Jordie, our potbellied pig. Jordie had an early career in entertainment and as an actor, but he has retired also. His room is in the basement and Jordie has become quite reclusive in his mature years. He is about 13 now and we call him "the troll in the basement." He is Dan's boy and is totally bonded to his daddy momma. Jordie just tolerates me. These are all the animals that usually live in the house.

Outside, we have three miniature Sicilian donkeys—Katie Blue and her yearling foal, Bonnie Blue, and a roan named Lollipop. We initially bought Katie and Lollipop as guard donkeys.

Why Bucking Bulls?

Donkeys inherently dislike canines and will chase them, so they are used as herd guards in some areas where there are lots of coyotes. Katie turned out to be pregnant and her foal was the first animal born at the 4B. More about that later.

We have two flocks of laying hens, each of about 25 birds. These chicken flocks are a mixture of brown and blue egg layers. They all have names and are pets. Their main job is to eat bugs, but we enjoy the fresh eggs also.

Then we have our glorious cattle. The heifers we bought to start out the ranch are the Red Baroness, who is our alpha female herd queen, and Lady of the Lakes, who is a very high-strung brindle. There are four female calves right now—Cali Rae, who is Lady's calf from last season, and the three amigos: Red Rosie, Africa, and Ebony Star.

Baroness had a bull calf last year, our first bull. We named him Time Bandit, and he is off at little bull school in Ohio right now. He will be bucked for the first time in fall 2007. We are expecting two more calves out of Baroness and Lady by the same sire, Priority, any time now. We are planning to work our way up to a breeding herd of 12 to 15 cows and are on a five-year plan to get to that goal.

So this is our cast of characters. You'll learn more about our adventures with them soon.

Chapter 2

Myths about Bull Riding and Bull Riders

There are many myths about this sport and the athletes that make it go. This chapter is for those of you that don't have much familiarity with bull riding. It will help to clear up some common misconceptions about the activity. But first, a primer on the world of bucking bulls and bull riding. Bull riding started out as a play activity that working cowboys participated in to unwind. The nastiest bull on the range got rounded up and the guys tried to ride it. Money changed hands over the outcome.

Dr. Eileen A. Schweickert

In the old days, the bulls were culled out of the herd when guys wanted some competition. Now the American Bucking Bull Inc. stock contractors directory for 2007 lists more than a thousand breeders that are involved in the business of raising bovine butt busters. Some of these folks are cattlemen and raise beef cattle also. Others are just in the business of working out bull genetics and breeding for the bucking arena. Herd sizes range from a few cattle to large herds of thousands.

As rodeo evolved out of these informal competitions and the wild west shows, bull riding was one of the "rough stock" events. As opposed to barrel racing and roping events, when you competed here, you flirted with getting your head knocked off or stomped on.

Gradually, rodeo events became more organized, competitive associations formed, and the money involved in these competitions grew. In the last 15 years, bull riders booked several venues that raised bull riding to the level of a standalone extreme sport. The Professional

Myths about Bull Riding and Bull Riders

Bull Riders Tour (PBR) is the most famous and successful of these endeavors. To compete in this arena is the big time for any rider or bull. And both are regarded as professional athletes in the sport.

Currently, the sport has the fastest growing fan base of any pro sport going. The average fan is middle to upper income, and both follows the tour on television and goes to live events. They buy lots of merchandise and like to travel to shows.

Many of us ranchers have small breeding herds and won't ever have more than 50 head on our pastures. We breed, buy and sell stock, and once in a while come up with a real powerhouse. And we have a blast doing it. Now, on to the myths.

Myth 1: Performance Enhancing Drugs Are Common

Most people think that this sport is fueled by Jack Daniels and other alcoholic beverages.

Dr. Eileen A. Schweickert

They figure that without alcohol, nobody would ever climb on bulls in the bucking chutes. This might have been the case before the era of professional bull riding, but not anymore. Too much is at stake to try to compete without a clear head. The competitive road is long and hard just to make it into the uppermost pro circuit. The bull breeding programs now generate monster bovines and you have to be at the top of your game to take them on. It would be suicide to compete intoxicated.

I have been impressed with how down to earth and unpretentious even the World Champion cowboys are. These men are gentlemen of the old school. They take their work and their fans seriously. They train hard, travel a lot, and like to spend free time on their ranches with family and close friends. Most of these men are working cowboys when not on tour, with hay to mow, families to feed, and mortgages to pay. These cowboys probably consume their share of Jack Daniels and Budweiser, but not while working.

Myths about Bull Riding and Bull Riders

Myth 2: The Sport Is Cruel to Animals

This myth comes from the mistaken idea that one of the ropes tied around the bull is tied around its genitals. This is just untrue. If you think about it, that would be downright counterproductive. The idea is for the bull to buck the arena lights out. Now, if you were the bull, would you even move if you had something tied around your privates? Come on.

There are two ropes that go around the bull. The first is called a bull rope. It belongs to the rider. He ties it around the bull's midsection and holds on, or tries to, anyway. The second rope is applied by the bull's owner, the stock contractor, in the bucking chute. It is called a flank rope, and it goes around the bull's hips. The testicles are free. Those testicles are worth a fortune, and no owner is going to do anything to make their bull's reproductive nature unhappy. Bulls buck because they carry a genetic tendency to do so when irritated or when something is on their back. Additionally, the bull does not like having anything tied around him and so the flank rope encourages him to kick, but it does not hurt the animal in any way.

The only other reason I can think of that people might think bull riding cruel is that spurs are used by the riders. Spur character is closely regulated by the professional associations in the U.S. so that no injury to the bull results from their use. In all my years of watching bull riding, I have never seen a rider hurt a bull. I have seen many a rider carted off to the hospital, though. This leads to the next myth.

Myth 3: Bulls Are Mean

A few of them are, but most just don't want anything on their back. Their owners can stand in a pen with them and hand feed them. There are, however, a few notable exceptions. The bull Reindeer Dippin is the first example that comes to mind. He doesn't like his owner, he doesn't like his pen, he doesn't like his trailer, he doesn't like his food, and he doesn't like other bulls. He has no travel partner as a result, and they have to feed him bottled water when he's on the road. He doesn't even like cows. But he actually has a reason for his foul attitude: He has been certified psychotic by a bull shrink. It's rumored that they may try Prozac on that boy. (This is a joke.)

Since bulls have to be handled quite a bit, it is actually easier for everyone concerned if they are not mean. Animals that are a handful to deal with tend to have short careers unless they are something extra special.

Myth 4: Bull Riding Folks Are All Ignorant Red Necks

Usually any generalization like this is untrue, and this is no exception. The folks involved with this sport are upstanding, hard working, salt of the earth people. They work hard for what they have and there are no short cuts in this business. To be a successful stock man, you have to have business sense and understand the science involved in breeding and raising livestock. You have to put in long hours and brave working outdoors in all kinds of weather.

Most of the people my age that I've interfaced with in the industry are college educated. This includes many of the bull riders. In fact, lots of these guys went to college on bull riding scholarships. Riders can make millions of dollars on the pro tour, so they have agents, lawyers, and brokers just like any other pro athlete. Some of the animals now even have agents.

This is big business in typical American style, with all the accoutrement. But there is one thing about this sport that is different. All the players in this arena keep a small head and a humble attitude. There have not been any drug use scandals that I am aware of. Riders circle the arena after each event and give out autographs to any and all comers. If you stand around a coliseum before an event you are guaranteed to encounter riders and stock contractors, and they will always talk to you. This is a refreshingly clean family friendly sport.

Myths about Bull Riding and Bull Riders

Myth #5: Bull Riding Is Only a West Coast Sport

It's pretty amazing, but the sport spans the country now on a professional level. This year, there are events in New York City, Detroit, and Minneapolis/St. Paul, as well as in all the classic western locations. If a city has a large sporting event arena, bull riding probably happens there. Our season runs late fall through midsummer, when there is a midseason break for harvesting time. Then the events start up again and run through the PBR World Finals, which are held for two weeks at the end of October in Las Vegas. The other professional circuits have similar schedules.

Typically, there are events held each weekend. Currently, the PBR Built Ford Tough events are televised and shown on Versus and NBC. Here in Michigan, we have two top level PBR events a year, held in Detroit and Grand Rapids. This is not really bucking bull territory, but it is good fan turf so the tour comes to town. The bulls and cowboys arrive from all over the country

Dr. Eileen A. Schweickert

to compete. This past year, an event was even held in Alaska, and after the season's end, an All Star Event was held in Hawaii.

We have not met any other bull breeders up this far north in Michigan but there are other folks in the state down south of us. When you look at the breeder's catalog, it is amazing how widespread this industry has become. Most of the large operations are still out west on the range. Texas, however, is probably the center of the bull business, the area around Stephenville, in particular. I think that anywhere you live, though, if people ask what you do for a living and you say that you are a bull rider, or you raise bucking bulls, you're going to have a bit of explaining to do.

Chapter 3

Heifers on Board

Did you know that you can arrange to ship cows through the Internet? Yep, you sure can. We found that out in the course of figuring out how to get our new heifers from Cleveland, Ohio to our ranch in northern Michigan. We ended up doing things in a much more complicated way, because at the 4B we figure complexity means fun. And fun is what we live for! The higher the complexity, the more fun the task. This is a 4B principle.

For starters, the seller made arrangements for another rancher to haul our heifers Lady of the Lake and Red Baroness as far as Kalamazoo, Michigan, which is about 150 miles south of our ranch in Mesick. We were able to borrow a livestock trailer, so along with a rented truck to pull it, we set out on our mission to collect our cows. Sounds simple. But nothing is ever as simple as it seems on first pass. This is another 4B principle: If something can go wrong, it most likely will. In fact, you can just about bet it will.

Our first problem involved the rental truck. We rented a truck because our ranch truck is old, and we didn't want to run into problems with two potentially surly, pregnant cows on board. However, the battery in the rental truck turned out to be a clunker, which Dan had to jump to get started. Of course, nobody was on hand at the rural rental outfit to deal with this issue; the keys had just been left in the truck and we had cows waiting. There seemed nothing to do but get her started and then not turn off the ignition till the adven-

Heifers on Board

ture was over. All potty stops, meals, etc., had to be made with the engine running. Okay, we can do that.

Fortunately, we made it to Kalamazoo without any other problems surfacing and found the ranch we were looking for. Our heifers were in a small corral. We backed up the trailer and Dan and the other rancher set about loading them up. Now, when Dan had initially looked these girls over, they were in a large pasture with lots of other cows. Though they were not hand gentle, they had seemed mellow enough. They calmly stood around, munching grass and flicking flies with their tails. They were girls, after all, not bulls. They were pregnant, however.

Next problem: Cows don't like change. They did not seem to think getting into the trailer was going to be a good move. When Dan and the other rancher began to try to herd them into the trailer, horns started to fly, hooves lashed out, and in seconds, a whopper dust cloud filled the air. One minute, they'd be heading towards the back of the trailer and it looked like all was going nicely. The next, Dan was running and scrambling over the corral rail with both cows on his tail, steam blasting out their nostrils.

Those heifers clanged and banged and snorted and bellowed, but finally both got on board. Since it was a warm, sunny day, we barreled down the highway for home so we could get the heifers out of that trailer as quickly as possible. We did have to make one stop at a rest area for the humans on the return trip, though. While waiting for Dan and monitoring the running truck, I decided to peek in the trailer window and see what our precious cargo was up to.

I stepped up onto the trailer hitch, shaded my eyes against the sun, and peered in. Lady was standing at the opposite end of the trailer, but when she saw my beady, little eyes peering in at her, she hauled off, charged, and hit the front of trailer where I was standing with as much speed as she could muster. I went

Heifers on Board

flying off my perch to the amusement of the guy parked next to us in his RV. The whole trailer rocked back and forth, and the noise of her head making contact with the side of the metal trailer sounded as though a collision had just occurred on the interstate.

Dan, ambling back from the visitor's center, got there just in time to see me go flying, watch the trailer rock and roll, and hear the racket. He decided against opening the side hatch to offer the heifers up a nice, cool drink of water. They weren't acting as if they were dying, and we figured that thirsty cows were better than pissed off cows, loose at the rest stop or running down the interstate.

We piled back into the beater rent-a-truck and made for home. We pulled up to our front pasture, opened the trailer door, and our proud gals came thundering out. They raced across the pasture and stood looking at us from as far away as they could get. Then they set about exploring this neat, new place, but were careful to keep a full pasture length between them and us for the next week or so.

Trailering is not always this smooth. We tried three times this summer to corral and load our heifer calf, Cali Rae, and little donkey, Bonnie Blue, to separate them from their moms for weaning. They won the contest 3-0. We ended up having to run a fence through the pasture and fence wean. Cali Rae would just not load.

On the first attempt, we easily locked Cali and Bonnie in the catch pens after dinner one night. We backed up the trailer. We got positioned and Cali ran right into the trailer, slick as can be, but she was so fast that she ricocheted back out before Dan could get the door shut. Cali Rae bounded in and out three times.

On her third trip, Cali spotted a six-inch gap between the fence and the side of the catch pen and shot through that hole. She slithered along the eight-foot slit and out free into and across the pasture. Evidently, cows do not have collar bones and can collapse themselves sideways like cats. At least Cali Rae can.

Heifers on Board

We boarded that hole up, but on our second try at loading her, Cali did the same thing. Each time Dan tried to shut her in the trailer, she calmly just pushed him out of the way. Then Cali found another gap between the two sides of the catch pen. A space we thought was too small for her to fit through was just big enough for Cali to escape. Bonnie followed her lead and off they went, free again.

The last try, there were no gaps anywhere that were bigger than a garden snake could slide through. It didn't matter to Cali. This time, she knelt down, stuck her head and shoulders under the bottom rung of the catch pen rail, stood up, and moved the entire catch pen about 10 feet. Cali sprung the whole pen, and she and Bonnie danced off again.

This time, Cali circled the pasture and came back and stood in front of me. She bucked her way around in a tight 360 degree circle. "Bring it on!" she said. Then Cali calmly walked away to join the rest of the herd. She never once acted spooked.

Dr. Eileen A. Schweickert

I thought that Cali would be skittish about eating in the catch pen after the first try, but she'd saunter in there each evening absolutely unconcerned when I'd call her and latch the gate closed. She'd eat and then wait to see what we had in store. She knew she could beat us. We can't wait to breed a bull out of this girl.

Chapter 4

Bafler's Syndrome

It was time for another visit to the doctor at the University of Michigan. He put me through my paces: I walked on my toes, I walked on my heels, he peered in my eyes. I babble, and once more he does the good news, bad news thing. Yahoo! No new symptoms. My wacky rehab program continues to yield improvements. I'm getting so strong, soon I'll be able to audition for the role of a new cartoon super heroine. But then comes the bad news. What sucks monkey vomit is that they still have no name

Dr. Eileen A. Schweickert

for what afflicts me.

We call it *relapsing remitting MS*. This is the closest match, but the doctor really doesn't think that what I have is MS. I told him I need a name in order to wrestle with the situation. He shrugged and looked cute. I knew he'd cough a diagnosis up if he could. I left the big hospital on the hill, depressed AGAIN.

Then, over coffee at Zingerman's Coffeehouse, inspiration hits. I've got it! I'll name my own syndrome. Until medicine can give me an appellation, my disease will henceforth be know as baffler's syndrome, because it baffles science and it baffles me. Now I can move on. Why didn't I get this brainstorm sooner?

When people ask me, I will have a nice answer ready. Otherwise, I have to spend an hour describing my sorry array of symptoms and deficits. A name is a shorthand way to communicate how you've been hit upside the head with a bat in the middle of life's game. My one remaining problem is that there is no international covey

Baffler's Syndrome

of folks with baffler's syndrome. Right now, we all sit in the shadow of isolation. There is a MS Society. There are groups for people who have had strokes, or have Alzheimer's, or Parkinson's disease.

I don't think the MS people will mind if I horn in on their groups. I've discovered that I need a club to belong to. I should start a new group for other people like me, people who have experienced catastrophic disability but don't have a stamp on their forehead as to a clear cause. We need a good, catchy name. Let's see. The "Baffled Babes." Nah, we aren't baffled. Well, not all the time, anyhow. Medicine is what's baffled. Ah, the "Baffling Babes!" That's better. Or the "Baffling Babes Council," also known as the "BBC." Hmmm, that's already taken.

Well, it's an idea in progress. If anybody else is interested, send me an e-mail and we'll get some momentum behind the concept. For the meantime, I'll keep horning in on the MS Society and I can still belong to the United Spinal Association. Time to get back to the ranch and more positive things. There is much to be said for distraction when dealing with chronic illness and chronic pain.

While I recount much about my experience with MS and life on the farm with humor, I think it is important to acknowledge that farming is hard work. And I realize that there isn't much that's funny about being ill. But humor, for me, has been a prime coping mechanism. There are lots of books devoted to the serious side of MS. This, for the most part, is not one of them.

Seriously, though, when you farm, you take on the responsibility for the well-being of other living creatures. Novices need to realize that the chores related to their care are not tasks that can be deferred. If you have the inclination to ranch or farm, even on a limited scale, I would strongly recommend visiting a farm for a working orientation as to what it really entails before you start acquiring critters.

Though most aspects of animal care have some

room for a certain amount of flexibility, each animal has to eat, be watered, and has hygiene needs and grooming to attend to. They need medical care, and love and attention. All these things take time, energy, and involve cost. My maternal grandfather was one of 12 children, and his parents were dairy farmers, as were my grandmother's people. I have other relatives that are livestock auctioneers, and my high school boyfriend's family raised pigs. All his extracurricular activities had to be scheduled around his chores; they came first. From these experiences, I acquired a realistic idea of what animal care really entails before I got my first big critters.

The good thing about this project, and why it is a suitable match for me, is that the tasks involved in the animal's care can be conducted on a pretty flexible schedule. When I started out, I walked with a cane and moved pretty slowly. I had to stop and sit between tasks. I would feed grain, then pause. Then I'd water, and again pause. I don't have to do any particular job at a set time, with the exception of vet appointments and things like that. And those don't happen very often.

As I have gotten stronger and better, I can complete more chores at a stretch. But I seem to have a fixed limitation of about five to six hours of time up on my feet per day. If I am up and about more than that, I experience an increase in leg symptoms and start to lose my balance and ability to walk. This means I have to be careful and creative in how I structure my days, and alternate the physicality of my activities.

I usually do chores in the morning, after getting my legs under me and some coffee into me. Then I work at my desk and do housework, sitting as much as possible. Frequently, I take a nap in the afternoons and then feed everyone again in the evenings.

Being flexible and not doing things from start to finish has not come easily to me. I am a very production focused person, and once I start a job I like to complete it. Yet I have learned

Baffler's Syndrome

to break things up into smaller steps and do one part of a job at a time. You do have to be careful, though, and not get derailed and have scores of incomplete projects unraveling around you.

I make lists and cross things off when they're done. I keep a schedule book and put everyday stuff in there, not just formal appointments. I have "to do" folders where I keep partially done projects so I can pick them up again. My desk is still a mess, but I know where things are. It is an organized chaos of sorts.

Chapter 5

Picasso and Dali

There is never a dull moment when you live with a pig. They are like children. If you don't keep a pig entertained and challenged, it will find its own activities. One cold, winter day, when they were feeling a bit of cabin fever, our boy, Jordie, and his cat, Rodman, decided that they would try their hand at painting. Both Dan and I were gone all day. When Dan came home, he went downstairs to check on Jordie and found the most incredible mess. He found no animals in the family room, and the downstairs craft room door was closed. But he heard noises coming from inside that room that sounded suspiciously like pig grunts.

He opened the door to an amazing sight. Jordie had opened a drawer that contained some craft paints in small, plastic pots. Rodman had pulled the paints out onto the floor, and apparently they somehow managed between them to open all of the paint pots. When Dan interrupted them, they were just finishing an abstract mural on the floor in bright, primary colors. They had also painted each other. Jordie was putting green stripes down Rodman's side as Dan came in the room. Rodman had blue paint on his paws and was swirling it around on the floor. They were not pleased at being disturbed.

I came home a few minutes later and heard all kinds of commotion coming from the basement. I went right downstairs. There I found Dan standing in the hallway, crying. He was worried that the paint might be toxic to the pig. And he had discovered they had pulled out all the large sheets of stained glass that had been previously stored in his worktable and broken them into small pieces. We scrubbed all the paint we could off Picasso and Dali, and then I sent Dan upstairs so I could take stock and clean up the mess. As I picked through the remains of the materials that had been used in their afternoon projects, I discovered not only had they been into stained glass and paint, they also had smashed open about six pints of canned salmon and eaten it. Jordie had even chewed up some of the canning lids and left them around the room like wads of used bubble gum. He had also eaten a portion of a roll of steel wool from Dan's supply cabinet.

Unfortunately, I was in such a hurry to get the mess cleaned up before Dan could fully see the extent of the havoc that had unfolded, I did not take a picture of the mural before mopping it up. Moral of the story here: only keep water soluble paints on hand if you have a crafty pig. Also, install pigproof and catproof locks on the doors that guard craft supplies.

Dr. Eileen A. Schweickert

Jordie has also tried out his snout at electrical repair. One day, when he was a little piglet, I happened to notice that he had a black smudge on his nose plate. I know his dad likes his pig boy to be nattily turned out, so I attempted to wipe it off. The mark stayed put. I looked closer and found it wasn't a smudge but a scorch mark. This set me off on a search for what he had gotten into that could have burned his nose.

I located an electrical outlet that was just at Jordie's nose height. It had a matching scorch mark. It appeared Jordie had stuck his pointed little tongue into the plug hole and got both a zap and a spark. We immediately went about installing childproof plug guards in all the outlets at his height and hoped they would also be pigproof.

We found the guards worked pretty well. Jordie could work them out, but it would take awhile, and we would usually find them half pulled out of the wall and be able to replace them before Jordie could fully work them free. Sometimes we did find chewed up plug guards spit out on the floor, like discarded chewing gum. Once Dan even watched Jordie start to put his tongue into an outlet. Jordie must have thought the shock and burn were a nice kick.

Most animals have secret bad eating habits just like we do. I eat pretzels and honey roasted peanuts in the middle of the night. Dan loves cheese. He will get up at 2 a.m. and have a handful. Chickens are suckers for Styrofoam. I'm not sure if it's the crunch, or if it fills them up because it's indigestible, or what. If there is Styrofoam in our garage, our hens will find it. I am constantly finding chickens hiding in boxes and under Dan's workbench, chomping away on chunks of the stuff they have rooted up.

Pigs love rubber bands and latex gloves. They will chew them like bubblegum. Jordie has consumed unknown quantities of both. Sometimes I can bribe him into dropping his wad of contraband in exchange for Fritos or Twizzlers or a pickle. It has to be something really, really good or he won't trade.

Maile the beagle's illicit food of choice is major gross. Most of us would not consider it a food, but she does. She craves donkey turds. Maile is a poop eater of all sorts, which I think is common in beagles, but donkey turds are her favorite. I have to keep her out of the pasture or she power chomps them down. Besides her tendency to run off, her poop habit is the reason she is tied to a pole in a donkey poop-free zone when we are outside doing chores.

Cows seem to be exceptionally committed to good nutrition. I have not been able to induce mine to eat any kind of snack or junk. Not that I want them to, of course, but they always come to see what kind of food treats the donkeys happen to be getting. If it is grain based, I offer it to the cows, but they always spit it out. They have amazing dietary willpower.

I mostly try to give the donkeys carrots and apples for their treats. Sometimes I give them pieces of alfalfa cubes intended for rabbits or gerbils. They like those a lot. And they really like graham crackers and animal crackers. They all came to me addicted to them, but I try to keep these treats to a minimum because of the sugar.

It's a good thing they like slices of bread. I use the bread to get their deworming paste into them. I used to take the tube of the gunk, have Dan hold the donkey still, open its mouth, and try to squish the stuff onto the back of their tongue. Some paste would get into the donkey but most of it would get on Dan and me, and on their coats. Or they spit it out. It looks awful, so it must taste yucky, too.

At any rate, the donkeys are not big fans of the stuff. But they are supposed to have it about every six weeks. Yahoo. I read a tip in a livestock magazine that suggested putting the paste on a piece of bread, folding it in half like a peanut butter and jelly sandwich, and this would get wolfed down. I was sure that my donkeys would take one taste and spit

Dr. Eileen A. Schweickert

the whole mess out in a blob, but Katie, Lolli, and Bonnie thought the paste sandwiches were great. They clamored around me, making it hard to get only one sandwich into each donkey. If only all problems could be solved so easily.

Chapter 6

Waiting for Bonnie Blue

Whenever I want to fill a knowledge deficit, I tend to read like a vacuum cleaner sucks. Books and articles cover every surface while I am pursuing the answer to my questions. When we started to seriously talk about hobby farming, I started poring over materials about all aspects of farming. I got books from libraries, resale shops, yard sales, and checked them out of libraries. I read online articles and subscribed to a whole slew of new magazines. I'm always sure that the answer to my problem is there someplace.

Just as in medicine, you soon reach the point where you have amassed conflicting book knowledge about the subject you are studying, and beyond this point, without real world direction, confusion sets in. Trying to decide if my miniature donkey was pregnant, and if so, how pregnant, and when I did decide she must be, determine when she might decide to deliver, was all one great research adventure.

When I bought Katie and brought her to the 4B, she had been kept in a corral with a young male donkey named Drake. He was of the age where male donkeys typically become capable of impregnating a female. And the woman I purchased Katie from had seen him attempting to mate with her. So, there was a good chance she might be pregnant, which I figured would be a nice, little bonus for my donkey ranching experiment. So I set about waiting, figuring it would become obvious whether she was pregnant, or not.

Waiting for Bonnie Blue

Ha! Initially Katie was quite thin from having just nursed and weaned her previous foal. Months went by while I went about fattening her up. Pretty soon, she started to look fairly round in the middle, but still rather emaciated along her top line and hips. I figured she must be pregnant, and after about five to six months I called the vet to come out and take a look. When you have livestock, calling the vet is done very selectively because it's almost $100 each time that truck comes down the drive. And my vet has very reasonable rates. So you don't call for every little thing unless you are Donald Trump.

The vet poked and prodded and decided to draw blood, which is quite an endeavor. She looked and pondered and said that Katie is probably not pregnant, that her guess is worms. So Katie got some deworming paste and we waited for the blood test results. In the end, after the tests were all in, the vet concluded the pregnancy test results were indeterminate. She did find that Katie was infested with parasites, worms, in other words, and so we embarked on a several-week-long deworming project. A couple weeks later, I collected some of Katie's manure and trucked it down to the vet. Katie still had worms. More worm paste, and now some great looking pellets called Strongid X that I added to her food once a day.

After all this, Katie's belly deflated quite a bit, and so for a while I decided she was not pregnant. I felt disappointed, but reminded myself that I got Katie for a predator guard and that I hadn't really planned to breed donkeys. Then one morning, I looked out the window into the pasture and Katie appeared to have swallowed a football, and it was lying in the middle of her belly sideways. Maybe she was pregnant after all. So we began a period of belly watching that went on for about another five months. It is now about seven or eight months after we began the wait in the first place. But donkeys carry a foal for 12-14 months. And of course, we have no idea when exactly she might have gotten pregnant. If she was pregnant.

Katie looked too healthy to be growing a tumor, though, and so I decided to just wait and not blow the $100 on having the vet trot out. It couldn't be worms or a tumor.

In July, I told everyone I was convinced Katie would deliver in early August. August passed. September passed. Finally my husband started telling everyone who asked that Katie was going to carry this baby for four years. Then one day Katie's teats started to extend and her milk bag started to puff. I called everyone I knew, and then they started calling me back every few days, and still she didn't give birth. I slept with the window open so I could hear if any commotion occurred in the pasture.

Two nights we had false alarms. I was awakened by Katie's companion braying her head off at 1 or 2 in the morning. I tumbled out of bed, ran around getting pants on, slapped my headlamp on my noggin, and trotted out to the pasture to find the donkeys standing around. The cows got up, too, and came over to see what this weird party in the wee hours was all about. Nothing happened. Twice we ran through this whole drill.

I read all I could about what to expect and assembled my "birth kit" per magazine instructions. I called the vet to be sure I knew what to look for. She laughed her head off at me. She said to forget all the stuff I read in my donkey magazines. Katie would give birth without any assistance, in the middle of the night when it was cool, and I'd know because in the morning I'd walk out there, and instead of two donkeys there would be three. I still had my iodine and dental floss at the ready, and my chair out by the corral gate, but in the end, the vet was right.

On September 13, as I looked out into the pasture from my front window, after getting a cup of coffee and my eyes focused, I saw a new set of ears, on a tiny, little baby standing next to its proud momma. I threw the coffee in the air, ran outside before realizing I was barefoot, locked myself out at the front door, and danced around crying as I looked for some shoes in the garage. Not a peep had come from

Waiting for Bonnie Blue

the pasture overnight. Mom and baby were both perfect and fine, and happily going about their donkey business, just a little concerned at my hysteria.

Chapter 7

Chicken Rancher Maile

How hard can it be raising laying chickens? Most farms seemed to have them in the "olden days." Somehow, I convinced Dan that this would be a worthwhile endeavor for the 4B. I studied various catalogs and selected an assortment of types of chicken that appeared to be suitable for our climate. I surely never imagined that there were so many kinds of chickens to pick from.

I selected some Rhode Island Reds, Araucanas, Silver Laced Wyandottes, and Buff Orphingtons. These are all heavier, larger, brown egg layers, except the Araucanas, which are the "Easter egg chickens" and lay blue, pink, and greenish eggs. The heavier birds are supposed to be best for colder climates. Otherwise, I selected the birds based on what they looked like. I picked kind of a kaleidoscope of colors.

We decided to time our first flock with the break in the cold Midwest weather. We figured that by the end of April, we would be able to keep a brooder area warm enough in the garage, so we picked April 26 for our chick delivery to take place. Dan had rigged everything up for their arrival. We had feeders and waterers, a brooder lamp, chick feed, and wood chips. We got all this stuff at the local feed store.

Our chickens were ordered from McMurray Hatchery. The hatchery gave them some shots and shipped the chicks with some antibiotic additive to be put in their water initially. The

Chicken Rancher Maile

folks there were very helpful and instructed me to work out arrangements with my post office to pick them up on delivery day. I was amazed to find out that yes, they would let me come in early before opening time and pick up my day-old chicks. I was all set to call on "the day" to confirm that my babies were indeed there when the postmistress called me. Wow! Maile and I set off in the truck, through the snow, to collect them. Yep, snow. This was not in the plan but not entirely unexpected.

I had ordered 25 chicks, which is the minimum number you seem to be able to get from any of the chicken sellers. McMurray also gives you a bonus chicken with each 25 chickens you order. Needless to say, I was expecting a good-sized box. I figured the container must be outfitted with food and water for all these animals. Wrong! What was waiting was something smaller than a shoebox, with air holes and lots of cheeping coming from it. Maile was ecstatic with the package and immediately started trying to open it. We hurried home, and then the fun began.

Dr. Eileen A. Schweickert

My lack of chicken parenting skills became immediately apparent. My first dilemma was that we had an unseasonable cold snap and I decided that the garage was too cold to brood them in. So we turned our guest bathroom into a hatchery. I put pine shavings down in the new bathtub and we rigged the heat lamp from the shower curtain rod overhead. I unloaded the chicks into their new home. It took about eight hours for the chicks to stop shrieking. It's amazing how much noise day-old chicks the size of golf balls can make.

My beagle immediately feel in love with the puff balls and decided they were her babies. Since the chicks' first sight was of the dog hanging over the tub rail peering at them, and their first tactile experience was her licking them, they bonded to her as mom and continue to have that attachment to this day.

Now, as it turns out, if you want an easy start to chicken ranching, it's important to have a beagle. For whatever reason, beagles like to eat poop, and Maile is no exception. She

Chicken Rancher Maile

likes it better than steak. And one of the only problems you have to watch out for with baby chicks is that they don't get "pasted up," where their waste seals their butt closed and it gets backed up. This can happen as they get started with the whole eating, pooping thing.

I had absolutely no trouble with this "pasting up" because Maile was quite careful to check her babies as often as I'd let her in the bathroom to see about their little bottoms. So, if you are going to have a small chicken flock, get a beagle. If you are going to have a large operation, I guess you'll have to breed beagles, too.

My laying flocks have been very successful. I've lost only a few birds to predators or accidents. I sell their eggs from the ranch, at farmer's markets, and to one of the grocery stores in town. They are so good that I've gotten fan mail in appreciation for them. They don't really net us any income but they don't cost anything either, and the birds are also a key element in our fly and pest control program.

Dr. Eileen A. Schweickert

The birds have free range of the property and turn over the pastures, including the cow pies, and eat all the little goodies they find in them. We don't like to use insecticides around our breeding animals, and because of the chickens and fly predators, we have not had to. Fly predators are small insects that prey on the fly larvae. We get packages of them a couple times a month and release them in the pastures. With these two measures, we've been able to control the bugs without chemicals. The eggs are a bonus!

We have had good success with keeping our chickens laying all year round by letting them outside all the time and keeping a brooder lamp in the coop when the temperature drops below freezing. This keeps water from freezing inside the coop, and the warmth is adequate to keep the birds laying.

The coops are also heated by the composting manure and wood chips on the coop floors. I only remove this once a year, in the early summer. When the floor gets damp, or the coop gets smelly, I put down a fresh layer of wood chips but do not take up the old stuff. It piles up over the year, and during the winter there is a good, thick layer composting, and in the process, producing heat. This helps keep the coop warm. Amazingly, it is not too smelly.

Dan installed some vents in the coop that have temperature controlled openings. They open and close based upon the air temperature inside the coop. These have worked great. Additionally, each coop has a window that opens and a door that I fit through, as well as a chicken hatch. The hatch doors are open all the time so the birds have access to the out-of-doors whenever they like.

Our birds get a combination of commercially prepared layer's mix, cracked corn, scratch grains, and steamed oats. We also feed all the food scraps we have to them, and they get some more veggie scraps from our ranch hand who picks up a bucket full once a week when he does his volunteer stint at the local co-op grocery. When the snow breaks and the birds

Dr. Eileen A. Schweickert

are out on the pasture, they don't eat much feed. They prefer what they find and catch themselves out and about to what comes from the feed store.

Chapter 8

Laying an Egg

Do not read on if you are both squeamish and an egg eater—this will put you off your omelets.

When I set off with my laying flock, I had no idea that laying an egg was such a big deal for the hen. At the 4B, you can tell when laying is occurring. Only a deaf person could miss the event. My chickens squawk up a storm right through the whole business and then for about 10 minutes thereafter. I thought maybe this

Dr. Eileen A. Schweickert

would stop after the novelty of the experience wore off and they became experienced hens. No such luck. It's been a year now and the racket continues.

I asked friends that have chickens if their hens did this since I did not find it mentioned in any of my chicken reference sources. Nobody else seems to have chickens that do this. For a while, I thought maybe mine were just theatrical, but one day I happened to be in the coop with the nest box open when one of my Buff Orphingtons dropped her precious load. And now that I've witnessed the process, I think all hens should be yelling their heads off. All the time.

What I saw was shocking. The hen, Agatha, had her back to me. She was sitting on her little nest of wood chips and I thought she was asleep when I first raised the nest box door. Then she ruffled her feathers a bit and seemed to leave them puffed out from her sides. I looked up, and all of the sudden she lifted her little rump off the nest and start-

Laying an Egg

ed straining and screeching. Before my wide eyes, her vent (the opening the eggs come out) gaped. And my goodness, an egg was coming right at me. And it was seeming to emerge from the Lincoln Tunnel. I was given a good, long look into Agatha's innards. I think I saw her gizzard. I swear, as the biggest diameter of the egg was passing, and she was in full yell, I could see daylight at the other end, where she had her mouth wide open.

Then her egg slid out, her vent closed, and she quieted. She tucked in her pretty, soft, yellow wings and settled herself on her new prize. I was holding onto the side of the chicken palace and sweating in commiseration. Agatha went to sleep. I finished my business and closed the nest box door. I decided to let her keep her egg for a bit, after all of that, and come back and collect eggs later. When I went in the house, I told Dan about my National Geographic moment. We decided that the hens were entitled to make all the noise they wanted. He said to ask them if they wanted a P.A. system so they could really let her rip. When queried, they held a caucus, but voted to decline the amplification. They are "all natural, free-range chickens," after all.

Now Maile is not the only one around here that hides eggs. Every once in awhile, various hens decide to play tricks on me and try to keep their eggs in places other than the nest boxes. Sometimes they dig holes in the wood chips on the coop floors and lay there for a time. One hen will start this, then others will add their eggs in that place. I collect them all, so I am not sure whether they are trying to hide them from me.

When we are not in snow season and the hens are ranging about, they will pick more out-of-the-way places to stash their eggs. Last summer, I left a good part of the back chicken pasture wild and did not mow it. The plants and weeds grew shoulder-high. The chickens hollowed out passages down at their level, and some of the girls would pick places out in their wild land to lay.

Laying an Egg

At first, this was a hassle. It was hard to locate the eggs in all the brush, and I didn't want to be collecting old eggs since I'm sure they wouldn't taste too great. They don't look any different from the fresh ones, so it's impossible to tell them apart. I either had to comb the yard, getting scratched up in the process, or chuck any eggs I found, unsure of their freshness.

Then I got the idea of trying my egg-sniffing beagle out as an egg finder. It worked wonderfully. I'd turn Maile loose in the yard and would simply have to follow her to where she'd stop; there would be an egg. The only trick was that I had to be quick enough to pick the eggs up before she ate them. Maile quickly got the hang of the game, though, and realized I wanted to collect the treasures, and would just take me to them and show me where they were.

Dan recently located a major stash of more than a dozen blue eggs in between the stacked hay bales out back. Some of the ranging Aracanas

Dr. Eileen A. Schweickert

that lay the blue eggs have been squashing up between the big 500-pound rolls and dropping their eggs in that spot for a good while now. Another Araucana had been laying eggs inside an old car bumper that was resting against a shed until a new purpose for it could be found. I guess one of the drawbacks to having free range chickens is that they do range and can put their eggs anywhere. Thank goodness they are creatures of habit and mostly lay in their nest boxes like they are supposed to.

Chapter 9

Breakfast in Bed

Mice, moles and voles are the farm pests that keep barn cats employed. Our orange tom cat, Tiki Teasdale, happily took on the job of rodent control when we moved to the ranch. He didn't really have the constitution for the job but he made up for his physical limitations with enthusiasm and smarts.

We noticed soon after we had adopted Tiki that he had limited wind and endurance. He loved to run, but when he did so, he quickly became exhausted. His lips would turn blue and he would lie down and pant like a dog. From his symptoms, I think he had a heart defect of some sort. As he got older, he became adept at pushing himself just short of his limits and relying on his intelligence in his hunting escapades. We thought he would probably die young, but he surprised us by growing to be a muscular, 20-pound tom.

At the ranch, Tiki took his job as head of rodent control very seriously. He patrolled the whole property and all its buildings every day. He checked the chicken coops, the cow shed, and the feed storage buildings. We never had any problem with mice, and the voles that often tear up a yard were his favorite quarry.

Each day Tiki would check their holes to see which ones were active. Then he would lie down about three feet from the entrance to a burrow and wait. From a window, I was able to watch him work, and that cat could wait for hours if need be for one of those fur balls to step out. Snatch, and he would have the vole.

Breakfast in Bed

Tiki liked to go out when Dan left for work in the morning and he was ready to serve me breakfast by the time I got up. Tiki had a particular yowl that meant he had a present.

Jordie has torn the lower part of the back door screen to create a pet door of sorts. All the animals come and go through this as they like. Thank goodness it continues to keep most of the insects out. Many mornings I would awaken to Tiki's yowl and find him standing alongside my bed with an offering. Yum. Usually his catch was dead.

One Mother's Day, Tiki decided to offer me a special treat. He jumped onto the bed, where Maile and I lay snoring away, carrying a live mouse. Yowling with his mouth closed around the critter soon had Maile and I both awake. Tiki proudly set his mouse down on the quilt, then sat back expecting praise. Of course, Maile went nuts, the mouse began scurrying for cover in the bed clothes, and I began to utter the traditional female yips and squeals, which the sight of a mouse usually provokes.

Maile caught and ate the mouse whole! Alive! I calmed down and praised Tiki for his catch, but belatedly. He had hurt feelings and never brought me a live breakfast in bed again. Sadly, one late fall night, Tiki headed out for night patrol and has never been seen again. When he first went missing, I felt guilty and wished I had kept the cat inside so he would still be with us. But of all of us, he loved the ranch the best. His life may have been a bit shorter for living as a barn cat, but he sure had a blast. I guess I really would not have had it differently.

One night, shortly after we got Tiki, Dan decided to warm up with a hot bath after shoveling snow. While he was soaking, Tiki came in and sat on the side of the tub. His tail dropped into the water, then he patted at the bubbles with his paw. Next thing Dan knew, that kitten slid off the tub side and started paddling around in the warm bath water. Dan called me in and I found both of them decorated with bubbles and enjoying their spa treatment.

Breakfast in Bed

This became a nightly ritual for the two of them for several nights. Tiki would materialize when Dan ran the bath water and follow him into the tub. Tiki would swim around, then into Dan's arms to rest. Then he'd take another lap around the tub. Tiki's affinity for bathing didn't last into adulthood but he never minded getting wet. He went out on patrol in any kind of weather. Tiki was not at all put off by rain.

Chapter 10

The Grand Procession

When the land is clear of snow, I try to walk our property once a day. I check out the wildlife, make sure the pasture fences are intact, see what new thing is blooming, and exercise myself and the beagle. We rarely ever do our patrol alone, though.

If it is not during the time of day that Jordie takes his morning nap, he sometimes is up for a hike. This is great for me because I have a long rope with clips on each end and can clip

Jordie to one end and Maile to the other. Then I don't have to hold on to either one. The pig serves as an anchor for the beagle. Maile can't follow her nose on a rabbit trail over the horizon when she is harnessed to the pig. Maile acts as a motor for the pig, who otherwise would start to root stuff up in one location and we wouldn't have much of a walk.

As we proceed along, the cats pop out of whatever spots they've been in and join us. Sometimes we encounter them out in the high grass of the pasture or someplace else, or on the trail through the wild part of the property. Tiki liked to sleep under the camper in the afternoon. Pintail watches from the porch. When the cats see our processional forming up, they will run to join the crowd.

Next come the chickens. We have a rooster named Pirate that keeps a pretty close watch on things, and if he sees us heading off, he usually comes running with a handful of hens in tow—his harem—and off we go. Those chickens will plod along with the rest of us and hike

The Grand Procession

all the way to the far tree line and back. Sometimes I have to get Jordie and Maile to round the birds up out of the woods and turn them in the right direction when it is time to head back to the homestead. They think the woods are pretty interesting, but they are not actually on our property, so I try to keep them out of the forest.

There are turkey flocks, a herd of deer, at least one opossum, rabbits, and coyotes around, yet amazingly, we never encounter other wild critters on our explorations. I imagine it is because, once formed up, we are kind of like a regiment of cavalry crashing along through the brush. The wild critters all run for cover long before we amble by. But we all have a great time on our hikes and it is good exercise for everyone concerned.

During the warmer weather, I have my camper set up over in the wild area of the property. Maile and I like to sleep there. We also have campfires there and cookouts on the weekend. We have had all kinds of nocturnal visitors at camp in the middle of the night. Usually, they check us out rather quietly.

Our most frequent visitor is Snorty the buck. We see him almost every night, just after it is fully dark. He comes around the front pasture and we can frequently hear him snorting at the donkeys up there, hence his name. Then he stands behind one big pine tree and snorts at us. When I first heard that noise, I wasn't sure what the heck it was. It is a harsh blowing sound. From my description, Dan thought it was a buck, and then I spotted Snorty and confirmed Dan's guess as to the identification of our caller.

When it has been really hot during the day, we sometimes have turkey flocks come through, feeding from evening to just after dark. They are easy to recognize, with their chucking and gobbling sounds, while scratching through the brush. They come right into the campsite. It amazes me that Maile usually only fusses the first couple of times a particular type of animal comes around. Once she knows what it is,

The Grand Procession

she typically just watches through the camper screen and is quiet. She seems to have figured out that if she barks, the critters will run away.

One night, we were awakened from the middle of our sleep by a loud, horrible screaming sound. I had never heard that cry before but was pretty positive it was an owl. It was hunting and caught what was probably a rabbit. There were the owl shrieks, then a rabbit scream, then quiet. Maile and I were both sitting straight up in bed, hearts pounding, as we listened to this drama play out. Maile did start to make a ruckus and I did not shush her till I had gotten my bearings and assured myself that it wasn't us who were under attack.

We laid back down and continued to listen to the night sounds for a bit. I counted shooting stars, and then we settled down and drifted back into a peaceful sleep. Although we make good use of all of our land, we are trying to share it with the wild creatures, too, and to be good stewards in the bargain.

Chapter 11

Cali Rae

The first calf born at the 4B came on a cold, windy day at the end of March. The snow was all gone, but it was one of those spring days that would have seemed cozier had an insulating layer of snow covered things.

None of the reference books had been very helpful in terms of exactly what to watch for to know when my cow was in labor. Luckily, I'd delivered a lot of human babies in my time, and that experience, thank my lucky stars, did

Dr. Eileen A. Schweickert

translate.

We thought we were prepared, in that I had ordered a whole bunch of obstetrical supplies from the livestock catalog and we had them all opened and in a tub stationed by the door. This included everything from OB gloves, which for cows, go all the way up to one's shoulder, to iodine to dip the belly button stump in, nose sucking bulbs, and milk replacer powder and colostrum. And a big pile of towels. When I talked to the vet, I could tell that she was skeptical about the pile of stuff I had amassed. She tried to remind me that being prepared can only stave off so much birthing trauma.

I was this neurotic when I delivered human babies, too. If there was a problem, it always seemed to happen when I was on call or on the OB ward. Over the years, this has caused me to be a bit anxious about the whole obstetrical field. My colleagues found it a cause for teasing, but I did not think there was anything funny about babies.

Cali Rae

When I was in practice, my partner continued to deliver babies. I did not. It made me crazy whenever one of her pregnant patients was in the office and starting labor. All I had to hear was that there was a pregnant woman in the office in labor and I had instant diarrhea.

I started checking on my pregnant cows in the middle of the night about three weeks before they were due to go into labor. I had moved a garden bench into their shed. I would put on a snowmobile suit over my P.J.s, go out there and sit on the bench, and watch them while singing Hawaiian lullabies. I was determined to be a good caretaker and not miss anything. When you have but two of the darn critters, you certainly don't want to lose a calf because you slept through the ordeal.

As it turns out, there are lots of similarities between cows and people when it comes to the whole birth thing. The three stages of labor give off the same telltale signs. You just have to make a few allowances for the species of the mother-to-be. Now this momma cow, Lady, is a bit on the high-strung side, even for a bucking bred heifer. The first indication that things might get a bit dicey was that with each stage two contraction, Lady laid down, rolled full onto her back, waved her four legs in the air, and bellowed like an elephant. Then she would get up and pace around the pasture till the next contraction came.

Lady looked kind of cross-eyed, like she couldn't quite get a grip on what was happening to her, but her body language clearly indicated that she was not keen on the process. None of the books had mentioned this kind of behavior, but in my experience with women, this kind of carrying on usually meant that I was going to have a job keeping Mom calm through the delivery. I kept my distance, sang to her, and put straw down in the places where she seemed to want to hang out. I wanted her to have a nice, clean spot to give birth in.

Well, this brindle heifer mom actually plopped out her calf without a bit of trouble, however, Lady's reaction to seeing this bloody, mucus covered pile of ears and legs was not remotely maternal. There was no licking and drying and getting on to nursing. Momma Lady just kept bellowing and decided that smashing her head against the fence was a good way to distract herself from the whole awful, gory business. Lady continued to have contractions as she still had to pass the placenta.

I could see that I had a perfect calf on the ground, but it was not breathing. Now this baby's grandparents are Hotel California and Red Silhouette, and daughter of Wrangler Rivets and Super Dave. These are some pricey bloodlines. No way was I going to lose this calf. This is where things got really crazy. I decided to crawl in there under mad Mom. I figured she'd let me tend that calf. I just had that sense. If Lady went for me, my plan was to roll out, away from the calf, and pray Lady would stick with her baby. Luckily, my husband hadn't arrived home yet. He never would have let me crawl in there.

My instinct was right. It was a good call.

Dr. Eileen A. Schweickert

I got in there and cleaned that baby's face off, used my suction bulb to get her nose and mouth clear and get her breathing, dried her off some, and then covered her with insulating straw to protect her against the wind. I ran for the house and got more dry towels. I also wanted to give mad Mom time to try to get a grip and take over.

As I was heading back out, Dan pulled into the drive. With his help, I was able to shoo Lady away and move the calf into the pasture shed and out of the elements. Then we gave her about an hour-and-a-half to calm down, but Lady remained a basket case and would not let the calf nurse. Each time the bitty baby got close, Lady would kick her away. That calf tried and tried, but the mom was just too crazed to settle into the experience. Finally, the little cuss just gave up and curled up on the ground to die. At this point, the alpha female in the herd, Red Baroness, had decided to come shove the little newcomer around a bit too, just to show the calf who was the pasture boss. This was not helpful.

By now, night was upon us. It was getting progressively colder, and the wind was picking up. The calf had nothing yet to eat, and it was critical that the baby get the premilk, or colostrum, within a short time after birth. So we decided to steal away the precious calf and let them try again in the morning. First, we had to chase Lady off. Dan bounced a rope off Lady's shoulder and we thought she had taken off across the pasture. We grabbed the calf, set her in a cart, and began to head for the gate and the house.

At this point, we heard "look out!" yelled from a car heading down the road along the pasture fence. We both looked up to see that Lady had come around the shed and was now bearing down on us at full tilt, her horns down, bucking up her back feet as high as the shed roof. She was still bellowing away, but she'd begun to get hoarse and was sounding a lot like Darth Vader. We dropped the cart and employed a move from bullfighting 101—we each peeled off in a different direction. Lady couldn't decide which of us she hated most, so she stopped a minute to think about whom to chase down. In the meantime, we made our exit and neither of us got freight trained.

As Lady was studying the matter, Dan roped her and quickly double tied her to the shed supports. He kept her secure, she went about trying to kick the shed to pieces, and I made off with the calf. Slobber was hanging all over Lady's face by this time, her eyes were bloodshot and bulging. I left Dan battling this demoness, and I dragged the cart towards the house and the warming pen.

When I got almost to the house, I made the mistake of looking back to see how Dan was succeeding in getting himself cut loose from his 1,300-pound crazed catch. Before he detached our Mother of the Year from the shed, he wisely decided he'd best have something between him and Lady as a bit of a safety barrier. While Dan let the rope out, he climbed inside the bale feeder, figuring he'd be safe there as he worked the rope off Lady's horns. When I looked up, I saw Dan and the bale feeder tipped up on end, zooming across the pasture. I was going to run in and call 911, but then I heard the old man yell out "Yahoo! I love this job!" as they scooted by. I decided not to look again unless I heard screams join the racket that this batty cow was making.

Eventually, Dan joined me with the calf. He was a bit dirty and had a tear or two in his jeans, and some straw in his hair, but he was intact bodily. Lady was still yelling away out front. Although it continued to be noisy, things finally started to settle down. We got that calf nursing on reconstituted colostrum and milk replacer from the obstetrical kit. The next morning, mad Mom had morphed back into the placid cow we recognized as our Lady of the Lake, and all was well in the pasture. The sun was shining, birds were singing, and Lady let our newest addition, whom we named Cali Rae, nurse. She lovingly licked and nuzzled the newborn and was the image of doting motherhood.

When our next mom went into labor a week

Dr. Eileen A. Schweickert

later, we girded ourselves with a new and improved battle plan, but Red Baroness just laid down on the manure pile, uttered one grunt, and pushed out her little bull calf. Baroness licked him dry, and got him up and fed, as though she was demonstrating perfect technique on an instructional video for other first time moms on The Learning Channel. We humans had absolutely no part in the whole deal. Not one thing in the OB kit got used. We didn't even dip that belly button. Figures, don't it?

Chapter 12

Bloody Rooster

Not all my endeavors at the 4B have been clear successes. I have had trouble keeping my laying flocks clear of roosters. I ordered sexed hens each time I sent for chicks, but the first batch included two roosters. Fortunately, I was able to find a home for them elsewhere. My second bunch had five boys in the batch. My husband and I agreed that we would eat them, but one has turned out to be an absolutely spectacular fellow, so he lives on.

Dr. Eileen A. Schweickert

This bird's name is Connie, and for the first several months, I was convinced he was deformed. His head looked like it had been shut in a door and squished sideways. Well, low and behold, he is supposed to look that way. He is some fancy kind of chicken called a Golden Polish and his weird head ended up growing a sprout of feathers out the top. He is an amazing combination of bronze and black. He can't really see where he's going, so he is actually pretty mellow. Connie has a pass from being processed for the freezer because he is such a pretty boy.

Now the second of my roosters should have graced the Sunday table because he actually is deformed. His head and beak are malformed and twisted, and he cannot fully open and close his mouth. But he is the friendliest bird I have, and so instead of eating him, he's become my pet. His name is Pirate and he follows me around the ranch like a puppy. He also loves to stand next to Dan when he works at his workbench in the garage. We both go out of our way to make sure Pirate gets food and water, and as a result, we've foiled nature's selection process and he's hale and hearty.

Recently, I'd noticed that the tips of the upper and lower parts of Pirate's beak were curling and starting to cross over each other. If left alone, it seemed as if he'd soon not be able to eat or drink at all. We studied all our vet and poultry books, and decided to try and trim the tips of his beak back. Pirate doesn't mind being handled once you catch him, so I caught him and gave him to Dan, who held him while I covered Pirate's eyes with one hand so he couldn't see the clipper, and with the other hand used a toenail clipper to notch off the end of his lower beak.

It went just fine. I quickly repeated the process on Pirate's upper beak. No big deal, and when done, he could use his beak a little. Success! We decided to take just a tad off Pirate's beak each time to avoid cutting too deeply and causing bleeding.

A couple of weeks later, Pirate's beak looked as

bad as ever. We tried repeating the process. I took about the same amount off the bottom as the first time, but dang it, the sucker started to bleed like mad. I successfully nipped a bit off the top, and then tried to stop the hemorrhaging. I shook some Blood Stop powder into my hand and began dabbing it on the tip of his lower beak.

Pretty soon poor Pirate had a blob of gooey powder congealed into a dime-sized ball at the end of his beak, but blood continued to flow. The bird had been fairly patient with us, but after about 15 minutes, he decided that he had had enough. Pirate started shaking his head, which sent the blood flying. We decided to turn him loose and see if the bleeding would stop of its own accord.

We checked on him after a half hour and found Pirate eating and drinking in his usual fashion. The bleeding seemed to be about stopped, but he had quite a mess down the front of his normally white feathers. Pirate looked as if someone had tried to slaughter him and failed.

Bloody Rooster

Yet the next day, you could not tell he'd had a brush with death. His beak had clotted off, his hens had groomed him up, and all evidence of the fiasco was gone. Recycled.

The hens thoughtfully spend a few hours each day grooming Pirate since he can't do it for himself. It is very interesting to watch. One hen sits on either side of him and one hen sits in front, and they clean and preen all his feathers. Pirate sits and sleeps while they tend to him. I can't tell if it's the same hens that do this or not. Sometimes seed cakes in his beak and they peck this all out, too. When he was a chick, I used to clean his mouth with my fingernail, but now he has his ladies do this for him. He much prefers his hens to me.

Although Pirate should be going into the supper pot, he is so endearing that we can't bear to part with him (at least not that way). He is the most companionable animal on the place. He follows us around like a dog would. He comes out to help feed the cows and stands on the edge of the food bin while we scoop out

Dr. Eileen A. Schweickert

the feed. Then he hops down inside the bin and enjoys a couple of bites himself. Next, he pops out of the bin and follows along, out into the pasture to check on the cattle.

Our front flock (Pirate's girls) eat very little chicken feed since they range the pasture. We offer them a blend of layer mix, cracked corn, steamed oats, and scratch grains. They do not like the layer mix very well and tend to leave that for last. They are fed twice a day. There's also a brooder lamp in their coop, which we turn on when the temperature is below freezing. It keeps their water open and helps warm the coop.

This combination of feed, heat, and natural light has kept our birds laying all winter, and we have not had any time period when egg production completely stopped due to a full flock molt. The birds do their molting in a staggered fashion. This results in the eggs being laid all year round. I sell the eggs here at the ranch, in the local hardware store, and at one of the grocers in Traverse City. The egg sales just about pay for the chickens' feed. This helps offset the cost of keeping them, and is really a bonus since we have the chickens primarily for pest control.

I had no idea that I would find so much personality in these birds. Each one is very different, and I really love my chickens. They neither chase nor peck at me and are quite tame. All of them like to be picked up and petted, scratched on their breasts, and have their feet rubbed. Dan is now accustomed to me coming inside the house and sitting on the couch holding a chicken. I have names for most of my 50 birds and can tell the majority of them apart by their behavior and appearance. Some, like Pirate, come when I call them. I can't imagine the ranch without them.

Chickens are very vocal creatures and have quite a range in vocabulary. I can tell their egg laying calls from their fright sounds made when a predator appears. They also have a babble noise they make when they see the scrap food bucket, another for when I fill their feed pan, and yet another for when they are getting ready to roost at night. They have angry sounds too, and even some curse words when they fight. Chicken society is about as complex as ours. Who would have thought?

There is an interesting phenomenon I have noted that plays out across the animal kingdom. I used to think it was only a human trait, but it seems we all come across it genetically. It must be linked to something that is meant to result in the perpetuation of the species. Otherwise, I imagine the end result would have caused us to become extinct a long time ago. I call it the Us and Them Factor.

Groups of animals that are acculturated tend to view and avoid other groups with high suspicion. You would see this if you watch my two chicken flocks. Group one, the Fat Girls, are in an enclosed pasture. They can jump over the fence when they want to, and three of them do so regularly. Bandit, Roberta, and Reddy choose to forage outside their enclosure a good part of each day.

Bloody Rooster

When group two, the Chickadoos, were old enough to be allowed out of their mobile coop, we moved them from their initial location in the front pasture to a spot just outside our front pasture. They are now free to range the entire acreage, the road, neighbors' land, and the whole darn county if the mood strikes them. Yet, it was inevitable that the two groups would have an encounter before too long. And they did.

Each day throughout the summer, I like to float about in my swimming pool doing aqua therapy while watching chickens. It was from this vantage point that I was able to study an experiment in sociology. Roberta, Bandit, and Reddy would be busy pecking around the hay bales, when suddenly, one of them would spy a stranger bird coming around the bale from the other way. Both birds would freeze, and you could see their sparkly, little eyeballs flitting back and forth. The rest of each group would stand rigidly still, contemplating the situation. Then, as if each had seen a horror, both birds would turn and run in opposite directions while squawking up a blue streak. The Fat Girls would run for the fence and jump back into their enclosure, where their colleagues had mustered to see what all the ruckus was about.

All the Fat Girls would get into a big jabbering huddle and decide by committee to stand guard along the fence line, hiding behind clumps of brush and waiting to see if the monster birds would try to invade. They do not seem to be assuming an aggressive stance, so I'm not sure what they would do if the creatures they are viewing were to mount some kind of an offensive. Luckily for them, this doesn't happen.

The Chickadoos, when they spot the advance party of the Fat Girls, do the same freeze, eye dart as their initial response, then run like hell in the other direction. So no actual conflict ensues. Whew! That was close! They scurry off around the hay bales and back to where their coop is located. When they encounter others of their flock, they stop and jabber, filling them in on the strange, horrible, foreign birds they'd bumped into while out on their morning constitutional.

This whole process repeats itself day after day, all summer long. Fall comes and the weather turns cold. Still, there is no mixing of these two groups or any change in their attitude of suspicion towards one another. After the first truly cold nights and hard frosts, I did note one day while in the Fat Girl's coop, that somehow there was one Barred Rock hen in that flock. Now, there had been no birds of this breed in that bunch. For some reason, this one bird decided to jump the fence and move in with the flock of Fat Girls.

The new arrival was initially pecked at and had to eat last, drink last, and lay her eggs on the floor because the mavens of the nest box—Agatha and Agnes—declined her entry. But, she did not leave. She stuck it out, and eventually she gained full acceptance. I call her Beatrice, and she now has full Fat Girl privileges.

So it goes for all of God's creatures. The pres-

Dr. Eileen A. Schweickert

ence of a group seems scary and impermeable, but one-to-one we are able to see each other, interface, and actually find common ground. Funny to find that people and chickens, with our variously sized brain pans, are still so much alike.

Chapter 13

The Day the Poop Wagon Attacked

Donkeys are the funniest critters on four hooves. I got mine to use as predator guards, but they are so entertaining and so cute that I'd never part with them. I currently have three. Dan calls them "the three stooges." Mine are Miniature Sicilian, or Mediterranean Donkeys. If you want to use the long-eared equines as predator guards, you will want to bear in mind the size of the herd you are guarding and the intensity of your predator pressure when selecting your donkeys.

Dr. Eileen A. Schweickert

There are three sizes of donkeys. If you have large herds and lots of predator loss, or large predators, you will want to get mammoth donkeys, or at least standard size, and have a greater donkey presence. If you have less of a problem, miniatures will work.

Because we only have the occasional coyote or fox to deal with, and all our pastures are securely fenced, we decided on miniatures, and three have worked very nicely for starters. As our cattle increase, we will also add to the number of donkeys we run.

Donkeys inherently dislike canines, and unlike horses, will stand and even attack them when threatened. They are quite fierce—hissing, braying, snorting, and stomping. Once, when I was in a neighbor's barnyard, I saw a pet dog go into a donkey corral and barely escape death. The dog slipped in under the fence to follow its owner into the pen, and the donkeys all immediately went for it, kicking and trying to stomp its guts out. Luckily, the poor, little dog was able to jet back out under the pen rail

The Day the Poop Wagon Attacked

before getting its lights put out.

A female donkey is called a jenny. The jennies are very maternal and extend their mothering to the offspring of other animals. Katie, our oldest jenny, always stands outermost in our shed at night. Farthest back in the shed are the calves, then the cows, then the younger donkeys, then Katie. For the first three weeks after last spring's calves came, she slept standing up every night. On guard. She sometimes lies down and sleeps in the afternoons, but at night she usually does not sleep lying down.

Something to bear in mind is that donkeys get into everything. This mischievousness is a mark of their intelligence. They love to play, and mess with everything they can get ahold of. Mine love to steal my pitchforks, brooms, and shovels. They think the sled I haul the poop with in winter is a great toy, too. My youngest, Bonnie Blue, frequently tries to run off across the pasture while dragging the sled by its strap.

Dr. Eileen A. Schweickert

One day, when she was bored with just being a donkey and decided to help me haul manure, she got quite a surprise. I'd dragged the sled into the shed and started to load it with dirty bedding and waste. The strap was laying where I'd dropped it, in a manure-free spot. Bonnie Blue came wandering over, watched me for a few minutes, and then suddenly snatched up the sled strap and started to run.

I grabbed for her and missed. My quick movement in her direction incited her to really put out a burst of speed. As she hurled out of the shed, her back left hoof came down on top of the sled, which was dragging along behind her. She thought it was chasing her and trying to attack her, so she clamped her mouth down on the strap and lit out across the pasture. She was not going to be caught by this monster.

The other two donkeys saw her bolt and spied the monster chasing her. They immediately decided to rescue their baby cohort and off they zoomed after her. Round and round the pasture the three went. After two circuits of

The Day the Poop Wagon Attacked

the yard, Bonnie Blue began to pant. Of course, this meant she had to open her mouth to suck in air, and that made her drop the sled strap. The monster sled flew along till it hit a snow drift and turned upside down. The smelly contents flew through the air, and the sled came to rest.

Bonnie realized that she was no longer being pursued and stopped in the middle of the pasture to catch her breath. The other donkeys and all the cattle slowly crept up to the sled and formed a ring around it. Slowly, they inched up. As it wasn't moving or making any noise, they got brave and moved in on it, and then started to attack it. They pawed at it, nosed it, and punched at it with their horns.

Eventually, I was able to retrieve my manure sled and go on about the business of mucking out their bedding. I'm sure this will now be another one of those dangers that the mommy animals warn their babies about when they all lay down in the shed at night. This will be known now and forever more as "the day the

Dr. Eileen A. Schweickert

poop wagon attacked."

My husband has also had his share of moments with "the three stooges" as he calls them. They love it whenever a project brings him into their vicinity, especially since he usually has tools with him. When a project takes place within their pasture, the donkeys try hard to help. Dan, however, tends not to appreciate their efforts to assist him.

When Dan was building a shed in the donkey enclosure, they did their very best to be useful. If he set down a tool, they picked it up and carried it around. If he placed something in careful position, they quickly rearranged it, sure their concept of how the whole project should come together was an improvement upon his plan. After several hours of trying to work, constantly having to retrieve tools and readjust his materials, Dan decided to eliminate his pals from the immediate project. He took a roll of old snow fencing and quickly constructed a barrier around his work site. He was then able to work undisturbed. His three

The Day the Poop Wagon Attacked

donkey helpers were restricted to the role of observers from the other side of the fence.

Dan came in the house for lunch, bravely leaving his tools laying about since they were now safe from being stolen because they were inside his tidy, orange barrier. He made a sandwich and got a glass of milk. He came into the study, proudly telling me of his solution to the problem of too many helpers. And he wanted me to go to the window and look out to see how well his new arrangement was working.

I followed Dan to the front room to look out into the pasture and admire his handiwork. He took a bite of his sandwich and pointed out the window. Then he choked. When we looked out, we saw all three of "the stooges" busy inside the orange fence, in the skeleton of the growing shed. Each had an implement in its mouth. They were jumping about and having a jolly old time, knocking down posts and pulling up measure markers.

Dan himself started jumping up and down,

growling about what bad critters donkeys are and how we he needed about three fewer. They had quickly figured out how to lift the bottom of the fence and slip underneath. There they were, looking like three donkeys let loose at Home Depot. Tools were flying all over. They were moving Dan's tool cart around, and pushing and pulling shed parts all over the place. So much for that idea.

Donkeys have a bad reputation for being stubborn animals. This is a gross misconception. They are very smart, though, and are self-protective. They will not do things just to please you. There has to be a donkey payoff. This is a critical thing to be mindful of in terms of training. Now, I've never had horses, so I cannot compare the two types of equines. But from what I know about horse training, you need to do things somewhat differently when working with donkeys. There are good training and care references available that are for donkeys specifically, so if you are adding long-eared equines to your stable, you can find good materials for guidance.

The Day the Poop Wagon Attacked

My roan donkey, Lollipop, is very bonded to me. I've had her since she was about six months old and have worked her the most of all my three long-eared pals. She is very protective of me when I am working in the pasture. She recognizes me as the alpha critter and minds me well for the few commands I've taught her. She always positions herself between me and Red Baroness, the alpha cow in our breeding herd.

Red Baroness is a bossy gal. She runs the pasture and has challenged me a couple times, but has learned to defer to me. She can be quite feisty on some days, though. Lolli is always watching, and if Baroness starts getting close to me, Lolli comes and stands between us. She always does this. If Baroness makes any move in my direction, Lolli turns and shows her back end. This is the business end of a donkey.

A donkey's usual method of striking is to kick. They are very exact with where their hooves land and Baroness has been on the receiving end often enough that she does not usually choose to deal with the back end of a donkey. Even her big rack of horns is no match. She lost a front tooth to a donkey kick early on and has had a healthy respect for the pasture guards ever since.

The first winter we all weathered at the 4B, Lolli seemed to intuitively realize that I could not walk and hold my balance very well in the deep snow. At that time, I used a cane and sometimes a walker to keep from falling. When hauling straw out to their shed, it was too cumbersome to use these walking aides, so I stumbled and tumbled a lot. One day, when I was pulling the sled with a bale of straw on it out into the pasture, Lolli came up alongside me and fell in step with me. I was able to hold onto her back with one hand and pull the sled with the other. She kept me on my feet and out of the white stuff. After that, each day when I would start my trek across the snow, she would come and provide me with security. If I started to fall, she would stop and brace herself to keep me upright. Lolli did this of her own accord. My trusty assistant!

Chapter 14

Cowgirls Love Trucks

Sometimes I think this whole "ranch" thing is my husband's way of justifying buying lots of big equipment, vehicles, and machinery—boy stuff. If you look around our place, you'll see metal hulks parked in just about every nook and cranny that doesn't have a pine tree growing on it. A good part of snow removal involves moving all this stuff in order to get to the piles of snow that accumulate around each treasure.

Dr. Eileen A. Schweickert

What all do we have parked around, you wonder? When we moved to the ranch, we each had a car. We also had a touring van that we'd bought from the wrecking yard with the plan to repair the side. It looked like it had been can opened. The damage was the result of a rollover accident. Probably, it scooted off the highway during one of our ice storms. All the guts were good, and boy, does it have frills. It even has a motorized bed in the back. It's a real pig mobile. Perfect for touring Jordie around. He loves to travel, but not every vehicle is pig friendly.

We also have a large, 25-foot, aluminum hulled boat that we're going to refurbish and refit for fishing, all that fishing we are going to do in all our many hours of spare time. She's called the Queenie Eileenie II. She's out in the back pasture and currently functions as a giant rodent condo. If you're a mouse, its a wonderful place to hole up and be safely out of the snow. All it needs is a big screen TV and pizza delivery.

Then, of course, you can't farm without a

truck. We needed to be able to haul hay and straw, and other things around, and pull a livestock trailer. The truck we got initially scared the crap out of me when I climbed on board. I about need rappelling equipment to hoist myself up into the cab. Now I only scare the other drivers as I barrel down the road or maneuver about the parking lot of the small town superette when I drive it into town on snowy days. The truck is an old, three-quarter-ton Dodge Ram with a stake truck bed. It is quite the monster truck, and I've come to absolutely adore her. I've actually not hit anything with her except the side of the garage.

My vehicle isn't the only thing about my personal style that has changed since I switched careers. Gone are the acrylic nails, silk suits, and pumps. Nowadays I wear a Carhartt vest, ball cap, and muck boots most of the time. I generally start the day with clean underwear, but I confess that I don't always get my hair combed, (you can't tell once the ball cap is on).

Dr. Eileen A. Schweickert

I don't wear chaps and a flak jacket when I work. That attire would be for the bull rider. You can easily tell the riders from the stock contractors in our sport. The bull riders are the little, slim guys with lots of scars. We stock contractors are the burly folks with beer bellies and all our teeth. I was destined for this life by my build. I have never been thin. When I dress up now, I usually have on a cowboy hat and some fancy boots. Fancy boots are any that don't have manure on them. No more pantyhose, thank goodness. I spent my life searching for a career that would not require those darn things and finally pulled it off. It's one of the good things about this new, stripped-down lifestyle.

My absolutely most favorite article of clothing is my mad bomber hat. My husband gave it to me for my birthday last year to keep me from freezing my ears off. It's made of Gortex and is water resistant. It's a fitted cap that clips snugly under my chin. It covers my whole head and is lined with rabbit fur. I look like Elmer Fudd in it. It's wonderfully hideous, but it is warm. The cows like it fine.

It is important to wear gear that the cows like. A while ago, I made the mistake of wearing a cranberry red rain suit to work in one morning. Mistake. I don't know if it was the color, or the swishing sound it makes as I putter, but the girls were running and jumping all over the place till I at least took off the top half of the thing.

When you work with cows and want to be close to them, and have calm pens and pastures, you have cow clothes. You wear the same stuff every day and launder it rarely to never. I wash my winter outer layers once each summer when they're not in use. To be the herd boss, you have to smell like the herd.

There are some special skills you have to perfect for the barnyard, too. Blowing your nose without Kleenex is one. If you did have tissue in your pocket, it would be too wadded up to be useful. So you have to learn the old "blast the nostril clear" technique. It takes a bit of practice but works great. You just make sure you are venting downwind because you don't want blowback. Some things are always yuck. Your own snot is one such substance.

Another of the skills I have had to master is the fine art of peeing outside without an outhouse. When you do heavy work, you want to reserve your energy for the important things. Extra treks back to the house to use the bathroom are wasteful. So, you end up peeing where you are. This is not such a hard thing for guys, but for us gals it's a bit trickier; we have more clothing to move out of the way. And different anatomy. Plus, whenever you squat down, the cows and donkeys come to see what you're doing. It's hard to pee when you're being stared at, and when critters are trying to lick your butt. You have to learn to be nonchalant about when you need to make a pit stop and saunter off to a corner by yourself while the herd is engaged with fresh hay or the mineral dispenser. Otherwise, you'll have more help than you need.

Chapter 15

Black Gold

A qualifier for a life as a farmer is your affinity for manure. This is a deal breaker. You have to be able to deal with the smelly stuff unless you are Donald Trump or Martha Stewart and can afford to have others deal with life's more unpleasant details on your behalf.

If you get squeamish about cleaning a toilet or emptying a cat box, forget ranching. You don't have what it takes. Remember, the bigger the animal, the greater the quantity of poop. It's a law of physics. Cows are the all-out and hands-down winners when it comes to manure production. They are really just large stomachs on hooves. After all, they do have multiple stomachs. Cows produce about 50 pounds of poop a day per animal.

My cows each eat about five pounds of grain and about half a small square bale of hay a day. And much of that comes out the other end. I think most of you know what cow pies look like. Actually, they really don't smell too bad. My mom maintains that my smeller must be broken, though, so this might not be true.

I am very finicky about poop in my pastures. I clean my sheds every day. In summer I even police the pasture, collect most of the manure, and put it in large compost piles. This compost spends a season cooking and breaking down, then I use this great fertilizer in my gardens, and around my fruit trees and berry bushes.

My cows do not lay or stand around in their waste. They usually do not have any dirt on them. It bothers me to see dirty cattle. That is my one criticism of some of my fellow stock men like Tom Teague. Sometimes his bulls charge out of the bucking chute with dirty bottoms. He should be able to afford to hose those beasts off before they're let out. He hauls trailer loads of bulls and has plenty of cowboys working for him. Give one of those guys a hose and another a shovel, Tom.

Manure is not the only noxious substance you are surrounded by on the ranch. If you liked digging in the dirt and making mud pies as a kid, then ranching might be for you. Mud is not a substance in my neck of the woods; it is a season. It comes after winter and before spring. It features cold water and the color brown. When you work outside, your feet are constantly cold because you are standing in water all the time. Thank goodness for muck boots and thinsulate. And one's hands are dry and chapped because they are always wet, too.

Mud makes you long for snow to shovel. When

your livestock sheds flood out, and you are shoveling wet straw and manure instead of nice, clean, white snow, you want to be able to turn back the clock a month or so. And all the animals get grumpy because their feet are cold and wet all the time, too.

It doesn't help that this season coincides with the time that momma cows are in their last phase of pregnancy. They are heavy, and can't run and jump anymore. They have backaches because of the big tummies they are carrying around and they want to lie down all the time. And there is no dry place to lie down; everything is awash in mud and water. Naturally, they get surly. When I ask Baroness if she wants to be brushed, she just punches me with her horns. Lady tries to pee on me. Thank goodness they only have about six to eight weeks to go.

And then it will be spring, when green rules, all the birds return, and we can start sitting outside in the afternoon. There will be grass to eat and the little pig in the basement, otherwise known as "the troll," comes out into the light of day again. At the 4B, we know it's spring because Jordie goes outside to eat grass; the chickens, which prefer to sleep in the trees, move out of the coop; and calves arrive.

There are still other icky substances a rancher needs to be able to deal with. Slobber comes to mind. The only animals that don't slobber on our spread are the chickens. Jordie slobbers all the time. His slobber looks like foam and makes him appear to have rabies. Maile the beagle slobbers when she gives doggie kisses and when she begs.

The cattle slobber all the time. Yesterday I got a whole face full of calf slobber. I had to remove and clean off my glasses in order to see again. I have been encouraging my calves to become accustomed to me by lying down in their hay pile and letting them sniff and lick me. This practice is something I learned from livestock guru Temple Grandin. I lie down on my back, and the calves huddle close to me and lick me. This is how cattle show affection and bond. When you at or below their level, you are approachable.

Cali Rae decided to wash my whole face with her rough tongue. I was able to scratch her neck and face, and it was really cool. My face was soaking wet when we were done, though. I had previously cleaned up all the manure around the hay pile, so I was not lying in poop during this exercise.

The more tame my breeding females are, the easier it is to handle them and tend to their needs. I have worked to hand gentle all my females and accustom them to me being close. Ranchers with huge herds do not have this same opportunity, as they have too many animals to get this intimate with each one. But part of my endeavor is therapy, and so things are a bit different at the 4B. I expect my breeding herd to reach about 12 to 15 animals maximum because I don't want to lose this relationship with them.

Even large operations and feedlots have

changed their handling philosophies and now focus on calm and humane treatment. Temple Grandin has done amazing things to reform the industry and I have learned quite a bit from her research and books. She is a person I would love to meet.

If you are going to breed animals, you need to be ready for lots of yucky stuff. Birthing is a very messy business. This holds true whether you are dealing with puppies or cows. But most of the time, if you let nature take its course, you can stand back and not get too dirty. Critters usually can handle the whole deal without help. Just like women. Another lesson I learned in obstetrics transfers to cattle: the birthing assistant usually doesn't need to get their paws in there. Calm support is the only contribution one needs to make.

Let's see. We've covered dirt, poop, mud, slobber, birth yuck. If you haven't gotten completely turned off yet, you might have a career in farming or animal husbandry.

Chapter 16

Stomping Chickens

Now this story has it all. Death, natural disaster, and a bitter lesson. It will demonstrate exactly how stupid I can be. Remember, though, if you are reading this book in a "how to" fashion, you will probably toss it in the circular file after I tell you about this fiasco. The moral of the story is to let sleeping chickens lie.

A little knowledge can be a dangerous thing. In my reading about chicken ranching, I'd encountered accounts of using mobile chicken coops, along with rotational grazing schemes for cattle as a method of pest control. Of course, the mobile coops are filled with birds. I decided to give this a whirl at the 4B. And it was a way to talk Dan into letting me get more chickens.

I ordered up a second group of chicks and planned to get a prefab chicken coop on wheels for them when they were ready to move outside. Dan, however, came across a little trailer that had been somebody's hunting hideout. It had been gutted to just a box on wheels, with open out double doors on the back, a window, and a door. Dan cleaned it up, installed nesting boxes, and we had a chicken trailer. When they were big enough, we moved the chicks into it and they were happy, little puff balls.

At first, we had the set up sitting in the side yard. Once the birds started to look like chickens, we hooked their hut to the tractor and moved it into the pasture. We put some snow fencing around it to keep the guard donkeys out of the coop. For about two months this ex-

Stomping Chickens

periment looked like it would be an unequivocal success. Those chickens did a bang up job of bug eating. There's nothing they like better than digging through fresh manure for little nasties. They just about follow the magic manure makers around, waiting for the stuff to drop. Since our manure machines are very productive, it seemed like a great arrangement. But then I had to get cute. I took in some birds that needed a home. What are a few more, I figured.

Three of these were little, tiny bantam chickens. I called them Snowbird, Tipper, and Tawny. They were very tame and loved being picked up. Then I started putting them on the donkey's backs when I was out playing with all of them. What happened as a result is the birds stopped being afraid of the donkeys and began running right underfoot at feeding time to snatch their grain. You know where this is going. Yep.

Well, one morning, one of the big chickens got kicked in the head. By the time I got across the pasture to her, she was dead. Now, the donkeys hadn't meant to hurt the dang bird. Katie even cried a big, old tear when she sniffed the dearly departed. But the bird was done for, nonetheless. I put the dead chicken in a plastic bag and stuck her in the freezer to await burial by the 4B funeral director, Dan the Man. Some jobs are just "man" jobs, and this was one. We could have eaten her, but Dan and I are vegetarians.

I briefed Dan on the disaster when he got home and went out to do evening chores. Well, dang if the same thing doesn't replay. Only this time, it's my Snowbird that gets stomped. And that was all the death dance I could take in one day. I sat down on the coop stoop with my mangled bird in my lap and wailed. Dan came running, and after about five minutes decided my mourning period was over. It was time for the burial. I'd worked myself up to quite a tearful frenzy by now and didn't want to give up my smashed pet. So Dan gave me another five minutes and then I had to hand over the "gol darned bird."

Stomping Chickens

We held a burial. Then Dan hooked up the tractor and pulled the coop out of the pasture and halfway across the property, well out from under all hooves. What we didn't realize was that as soon as we opened the coop doors the next morning, those birds ran right up front to get back to their donkey pals. Well, heck. And come evening, they were unable to locate their house. So we had to move the coop back up front, but we put it outside the pasture.

This was just too much change for all concerned. That night at bedtime, only two chickens were inside the coop. The rest were scattered all over the place. I went to bed hoping the coyotes and owls would give us a break but neglected to think about one more wrinkle, the weather.

That night, Mother Nature added her two cents to the pot and threw a whopper of a thunderstorm. It rained about six inches in an hour. I woke up with the thunder boomers and lightening show and remembered that my little flock was outside all mixed up. I pulled out some clothes and my headlamp and headed for the coop. Dang! Only two birds inside. I spent the next hour scrambling through mud puddles and plucking up my sad, soaked chickens from all corners of the land. They were on the fence, in trees, in feed bowls, and a couple were asleep in the straw with the donkeys in their shed. Little by little, I collected all the birds I could find and lined them up on their roost bar inside their warm, dry coop.

After about an hour, I found everybody. I was absolutely drenched and covered with mud. I had to peel off my clothes and leave them in the garage because they were foul. I warmed up in the shower and fell into bed. The next morning, the chickens were all dry, fluffy, and in good humor again. After that adventure they finally seemed to grasp where their coop was located in the grand scheme of things.

The ranging flock is hard to button down for the night since they like to roam until the sun is absolutely set and dark is falling. There is no

Stomping Chickens

coaxing them into bed early so I can shut them in and seal them off from nocturnal predator attacks. As a result, we lost a hen one night to some critter that ate its tail off. I found the dying chicken huddled up along the fence by the front pasture one morning. Her feathers were all over the coop floor, so whatever had attacked had come right into the coop.

That night I set out to shut them in after sunset. I trundled out to the coop in my pajamas. As I approached the coop, the birds seemed awfully chatty; they were yelling and carrying on something awful. Three of the chickens had decided they would rather sleep in 30 degree weather outside in a tree than face a night with monsters invading their hut. They were up at the top of a honey locust next to the coop. When I looked into the hatch door, I found the cause for all the ruckus. Something with a long, nasty, ratlike tail was eating the chicken feed out of the pan.

I grabbed a long, PVC pole and poked the monster rat in the butt through the hatch door.

It whirled around and scuttled into the corner of the coop. It wasn't a rat, it was a possum. A great big, fat one. I got a rake and shoved the door open. Now several hens jumped down, and sensing they had reinforcements, they started to attack the possum. It held its ground and hissed at us.

I swatted it a couple of times with the rake and it skedaddled off into the night. Unfortunately, so did one of the hens. It took me another 20 minutes of running around, hoping not to re-encounter the possum in the dark, to catch that girl and put her back in the coop. She had decided to take her chances roosting outside instead of going back in where the possum was. I finally let her go roost on the trailer tongue and then was able to snatch her up. By this time, I had made such a fuss that I had all the cattle in the proximal pasture mooing away.

So now I was shouting, the chickens were clucking, and the cows were yelling. Neighbors must have thought we were on fire, or under

Stomping Chickens

attack by wolves or aliens. Not even my husband materialized to help fight the Great Possum War, however. Good thing it hadn't been a bear.

Chapter 17

Newcomers

Our first bull calf was born in spring 2006. We named him Time Bandit and he's an absolutely beautiful creature. He's bright red, with white masking eye patches and socks. He has red freckles all over his pink nose. While his half sister, Cali Rae, is the unflappable, calm, sleepy-eyed baby, Bandit is a tornado on hooves.

Bandit would rather run and play than eat. His favorite game is head butt. Mostly, he head butts Cali, much to her displeasure. Even though she is a week older and a bit bigger then Bandit, he knows no fear. Bandit also head butts his aunt, Lady, who usually tolerates this without much response. He'll keep bonking into her side and she just keeps eating her hay. It's like he's invisible. She pays more attention to flies.

Bandit's most favorite thing to take on is the wheelbarrow. He'll bash on it until he knocks it over. Then he watches it for a bit to make sure it won't play any dirty tricks on him. Then he starts in again. Sometimes Bandit gets so wound up that he head butts his mom, Red Baroness. This only happens once in a play sequence, though. She scoops his little butt up and slides him across the pasture. Then she drops him on his noggin. This makes him pause for a minute. Then he'll get up and start head butting the dirt.

If there is water in the pasture, Bandit's in it. He stands in the mud puddles and just splashes and plays with the water. He stomps in it, and you guessed it, head butts it. I can't even coax him out of the water with grain because he'd rather play than eat. Bandit was a scrawny, little thing initially as a result. Then we discovered that he's a sucker for steamed oats. When Dan added them to his feed mix, he finally started to show some interest in his chow.

It's amazing how different in personality each of our cows are. A year along in our project, we bought three heifer calves and brought them to the 4B when they were weaned, at about six months of age. These three calves all came from the same ranch in Illinois and have the same father, but different mothers. They are double bred Watusi in lineage.

All of these calves spin and buck, and are very high-energy animals. They are slighter in frame than Bandit and Cali and their mothers. They are quicker as a result. The first thing the new calves did when they were let go in the pasture here is to chase the donkeys. The donkeys had become pretty lazy and fat, so this will get them back in shape.

Ebony Star is coal black. She has horns and is the smallest of the new girls. She is dainty and moves like a cat. She loves to spend her days inside the bale feeder, eating and sleeping. I have seen her roll over on her back and stretch her legs in a double jointed fashion that I didn't think a cow could pull off. She is small enough that she can slip inside the slats of the hay bale feeder and then Baroness can't push her around. So that is where she likes to spend her days.

Rosie is the only animal we have that doesn't have horns. It is a good thing. Like Time Bandit, she has a thing for head butting. She is the most dominant of the calves and pushes all the rest of them around. She is very high-strung, but in a tough way, not as skittish as Lady. She has got the most amazing punk hairdo. She is a deep, red and has a bright red stripe down her back, and a fringe of bangs the same color. She looks like someone at the salon went nuts on her with highlights.

Newcomers

Africa is our one light-colored girl. She is tan with some white spots. She has great big, brown eyes and is the donkey buster. She gets pushed around by all the other cattle, but she is the one that fends the donkeys off the hay pile and keeps them out of the grain bowls. She is fearless. She is the fastest and loves to run.

When Dan goes out to the pasture, usually in the evenings, they all play "rodeo." He yells and waves his arms, and all the calves take off. They run loops around the pasture and see who can race the fastest. They stop and spin, and then tear off in the opposite direction. They jump grass mounds and run up and stop on top of the manure piles and buck. It is an absolute sight to watch these magnificent animals perform. And they love it. It has become our after dinner game.

The only time our crew seems distressed is when spring melt comes and it's mud season. Then it's hard to keep the shed floors dry and everyone in the pasture gets a bit crabby. If

Dr. Eileen A. Schweickert

we get a good rain on top of the melting snow, then things go from muddy to underwater. This spring it almost got to the point where we had to buy snorkels for all the animals.

Other than wet, the only other thing our troop doesn't like is snowmobiles. For some reason, they detest them. We live in an area where snowmobiling is a popular winter pastime, unfortunately, so they have to endure the machines running up and down the road during snow season. I'm not sure what it is that bothers them, but I think it might be the noise. I don't like them either.

Chapter 18

Mornings with Martha

Most people with livestock probably spend quite a bit of time watching their animals. Life with animals is like living within a National Geographic special. However, at my ranch, the livestock also devote a large amount of time to people watching. This is especially true of the cows. Cows are among the most curious animals that you could choose to cohabitate with. Mine are no exception. Cows move around the pasture whenever you are working out on the land. Ours keep tabs on us and supervise

Dr. Eileen A. Schweickert

whatever projects we are dabbling at. If possible, they like to stand at the hay pile, where they can scarf hay and watch us at the same time. If this isn't possible, they can switch to cud chewing and observing, as they can do this from anywhere in the pasture.

Sometimes when you're involved in a particularly boring project, the cows will lie down and chew and watch. At first, it can be rather disconcerting, always having several sets of eyes on your every move. But if you have cows, you will get used to being monitored all the time. You will also become accustomed to not being able to do really stupid things in private, like tripping over your pitchfork handle and falling into the manure pile. All of your many clumsy moves and less well-thought-out attempts at solving ranch dilemmas are fully noted, and you are regularly made to feel stupid. I have learned that humility is a consequence of tending cows.

This constant surveillance can be wearing, though. Initially, I thought I could retreat into the privacy of the house. I thought I was safe from their view when I was indoors. I was wrong! I am not a morning person, and mornings can be particularly filled with difficulty as I go about the business of waking up and getting functional. I thought that whatever occurred between my first and third cups of coffee was between me and my buddy, Martha Stewart. And since I could see her but she could not see me, thanks to the wonders of TV, it did not matter that my hair was uncombed, my socks didn't match, and I was in my old lady briefs and a tee shirt.

Then, one morning, in the quiet of my living room, I was spilling coffee and trying to cut out a recipe from the newspaper when I realized that Martha and I were not alone. I looked out the living room window and found my cows and donkeys lined up along the pasture fence watching Martha and me through the picture window. I ran and put shorts on. I combed my hair. They couldn't be watching TV! They couldn't be watching me watch TV!

But they were. I paid attention over the next couple of mornings and they did not watch the *Today Show*. But come 10 a.m., there they were, lined up and jostling for the best vantage point. They seemed to be ready to create centerpieces and fold tee shirts, and were no doubt hoping that Martha was going to teach their dumb, old mom to live a bit more tidily. Now I know that the only place I am really safe from their peering eyes is in the bathroom with the door shut!

Several days later, I was visiting Martha Stewart's Web site looking for a recipe when a message popped up on screen suggesting that I send Martha a note. I thought the poor person whose job it was to respond to this onslaught of messages might get a chuckle out of my story about Martha's two "biggest fans." So I dropped Martha a line.

About 24 hours later, my phone began to ring. First, it was a producer's assistant from *The Martha Stewart Show* calling to ask me questions about my TV watching cows. Within another 24 hours, the cows had an appointment with a film crew for video taping, and I had interviews scheduled with a producer. We would all be on the show live at the end of the week: the cows on film, and me on the phone live in conversation with Martha.

Talk about pressure! It would be bad enough if Martha was going to peep into my house, but my pasture! In the dead of winter. I prayed for a snowstorm to cover up all the fresh poop in the manure pile so things would look pristine and beautiful. My prayers were answered, and the poor cameraman was out there in knee-deep snow, filming the cows, while they watched Martha through the front window. He was intimidated by the horns on Lady and Baroness and decided he did not want to go into the pasture.

Come Friday morning, I was connected by phone and got my moment of fame chatting with "the real Martha Stewart" live on her show. The great footage of my beautiful gals rolled and the audience seemed to really enjoy the story.

We had all kinds of fan attention for quite awhile afterward. People all over the country called to say that they had caught us on the tube. I was amazed to find out how many of my friends and acquaintances were closet "Martha" addicts. She has an amazing following, it turns out. Even beyond the 4B.

Martha mentioned that she would have sent the cows each a tee shirt but she didn't have ones big enough for Lady and Baroness. So she sent them each a gorgeous cowbell. Now when folks visit, we offer each guest the opportunity to hang a bell on a cow. For some reason, we've not yet had anyone take care of those bells. They still sit on top of the TV.

Chapter 19

Turtling

One of my biggest physical problems is with my balance. Or lack thereof. Since this illness began, I have been plagued with the peculiar sensation that I am cartwheeling over to the left. Luckily, this is not constant, and it has improved over time, but it means that I fall frequently. As a result, I spend a fair amount of time on the ground. Hanging out in this location has it's pluses and minuses.

Sometimes I get hurt when I take a splat, so

Dr. Eileen A. Schweickert

I try to stay off ladders, steps, and other places where injury is most likely to occur. Aside from getting hurt in the act of falling, there isn't a whole lot wrong with being on the ground. I guess one can get a bit dirty, but that is what washers and dryers are for.

My mother-in-law experienced something similar towards the end of her life. She called the experience "turtling" (seeing the world from a turtle's view) and learned to enjoy observing the world from the vantage point of the ground. I think she had something, and I have tried to share this perspective. It is all about perspective, after all.

The world looks a lot different from the ground. The main change I note is that as a person, you feel much smaller and less significant with respect to the rest of the world. You see all kinds of things that are around you all the time but often go unnoticed. The sky, for example, is huge. When standing, it is above you, so you usually don't pay it much attention. But when you lie on your back on the ground

Turtling

and look up, the sky is all that you see. When you watch the clouds skid by, you can tell how fast the wind is blowing at their level high in the atmosphere.

The plant world is also more vivid and detailed when you are looking at everything from ground level. My mother-in-law mostly enjoyed her luscious garden during her "turtling" episodes. I don't have a garden like hers, but I have discovered that there is a whole world of tiny plants, some with delicate, detailed, little flowers that live in our lawn. I never realized they were there. If you land under a tree when you flop, watch the birds for a bit. From the ground, looking up, it is quite a show.

My first reaction after a spill is to do a body survey and assess the physical damage. This is probably a carryover from too many trauma triage drills over the course of my medical career. Next, an acute wave of embarrassment passes over, along with amazement at my clumsiness and lack of grace. This washes away with the realization that whatever my ungraceful move was, it was unobserved by any other human.

Over time, I experience these feelings less. I think this whole illness thing has, to an extent, been an exercise in humility. And perhaps my opinion of how big and important a role I occupy in the world has undergone a shift. Now, I lie down on the ground sometimes for the view and the sense of peace it brings.

My calves have gotten used to me lying down with them on the hay pile. I love to look them over from this perspective. They are gorgeous creatures. They like to cuddle, and they will since I am down on their level. Mostly, though, they just lay in community, chew their cuds and accept me as a member of the herd. Cattle and most animals have a greater capacity to just be, remaining quietly still. I am learning how peaceful that can be. And how healing that peace is.

I have previously related the story of Cali Rae's birth. Her first night was spent in a warming pen, with Dan and I taking shifts at two-hour intervals, teaching her to nurse. We mixed and fed her reconstituted colostrum since she had not yet gotten this from her mom. Cali has a very long nose, and the various nipples we had did not hit her palate correctly to stimulate her sucking reflex, so we had a bit of a struggle getting her going. Dan discovered that if he laid the bottle in his hand, and used his fingers as an extension of the nipple, he could tickle her palate and this would get her to suck. She would then catch the nipple and latch on.

Cali was very hungry, and once she figured out how to get the milk, she clamored for it greedily. After a bottle, she would be overcome with a burst of playful energy. Her legs were still wobbly and she had no control over them at that point. Cali would try to buck and spin in a circle, and would end up in a heap in the straw. She was literally bucking before she took her first steps. We would help Cali up again and play with her for 10 or 15 minutes. Then she would be exhausted and lie down and fall asleep.

After the 2 a.m. feeding and play session, I decided to lie down in the straw with her. She curled up hard against me, put her head on my chest, and drifted off. Ever so often, she would partially waken, nuzzle my neck and face, then press herself to me and, reassured, fall back asleep. I could feel the animal's heartbeat next to mine and smell her milk breath in my face. Snuggled together, we were toasty warm. While Cali was sleeping, I was able to explore the wonder of her gorgeous calf body. The details of her coat, her perfect little hooves and a peek at what her tongue and teeth looked like. What an amazing creation!

The next morning, we turned her back out in the pasture and her mom had calmed down. Cali had learned how to latch on, so within an hour, they were successfully nursing and all was well. Cali Rae had no confusion about who her mother was or where she belonged. But both Dan and I had the blessing of our one night, curled up on the ground with that wonderfully beautiful creature.

Conclusion

If this book was an episode of *The Roy Rogers Show*, it would now be time for "Happy Trails to You" to play. I'm sure I could think of more tales to tell about the 4B Ranch, but the best and funniest have been set down here. My transformation from career woman to professional poop scooper is described in all it's glory, or lack thereof. I know that what happened to me happens to other people every day. Many people are forced to deal with major lifestyle changes due to illness or injury. My goal for

Dr. Eileen A. Schweickert

this book is to share the essence of what has worked to help me adjust and cope, because I think it might help others.

While I doubt that anyone else will resort to my ranching "treatment," I hope my story encourages others who have had to give up a job because of illness to find new ways to use their talents. Find a pursuit that fits your needs and occupies your mind, and you can be successful at overcoming the challenges life presents you.

It has been three years since my career change. As I bring this collection of tales to a close, I am waiting for my second crop of calves to drop. They should be born any day now. Our breeding program is going so well that I expect we will have our first animals up for sale next year. And my health has continued to improve. I can walk independently on most days. The integrated pain control approach I am using has modulated my pain to the point that it is not ruling my life anymore.

Conclusion

Some of these improvements have come because I have accepted my limitations. I have accepted that my medical practice is over. I have retired my licenses and moved on to tackle new projects. This is a huge loss. But I've grieved it and recovered. I am finding new ways to use my education and skills that accommodate my disabilities. Some days are harder than others, but when the times get tough, I've learned to cowgirl up.

Mahalo

I close this book with a warm "mahalo" to Mrs. Funai, my first writing critic. When I was a student at Waialua High and Intermediate School in Waialua, Oahu, Hawaii, she taught me the art of storytelling.

About the Author

Eileen A. Schweickert grew up a military brat, studied at the Manoa campus of the University of Hawaii, and went to medical school in California. Dr. Schweickert taught the next generation of doctors, climbed the ladder of academia and sat on the Board of Directors of the American Medical Women's Association.

Later, she settled into being the small town doctor she always wanted to be. But her rewarding career in family medicine in Northern

Dr. Eileen A. Schweickert

Michigan was cut short due to a nasty disease called multiple sclerosis.

Sensing that change was necessary to regain mental and physical health, she and her husband bought a plot of land to begin their retirement dream early—hobby ranching bucking bulls.

BMS

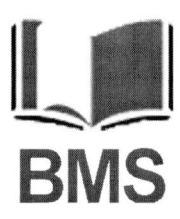

BookMarketingSolutions.com

Order Form

For additional copies of *Funny Farm*, please fill out the following information or visit the publisher's Web site:

www.ReadingUp.com

Discounts are available for bulk orders and to bookstores, libraries, and other retailers.

Fax orders: (231)929-1993
Telephone orders: (231)929-1999
E-mail orders: sales@BookMarketingSolutions.com
Postal orders: BMS
10300 E. Leelanau Court
Traverse City, MI 49684

Please send _____ **copies of** *Funny Farm* at $14.95 each. I understand that I may return any of them for a full refund–for any reason, no questions asked.

Name: _____
Address: _____
City: _____ State: _____ Zip: _____
E-mail address: _____
Phone (in case we need to contact you) _____

Sales Tax: Please add 6% for products being shipped to Michigan addresses.

Shipping by air:
US: $5.00 for the first book and $0.50 for each additional book.
International: $10.00 for the first book and $5.00 for each additional book (estimate).

TOTAL $ _____

Payment: Check   Money Order
Credit Card: Visa   MasterCard   Discover   AmEx

Card Number: _____
Name on Card: _____ Exp. Date: ____/____
Billing Address on Card if different than shipping address: